FUELLED FIT AND FIRED UP

To Andy
Unleash Your Roar!

FUELLED FIT AND FIRED UP

UNLEASH THE POWER OF A HEALTHY LIFE

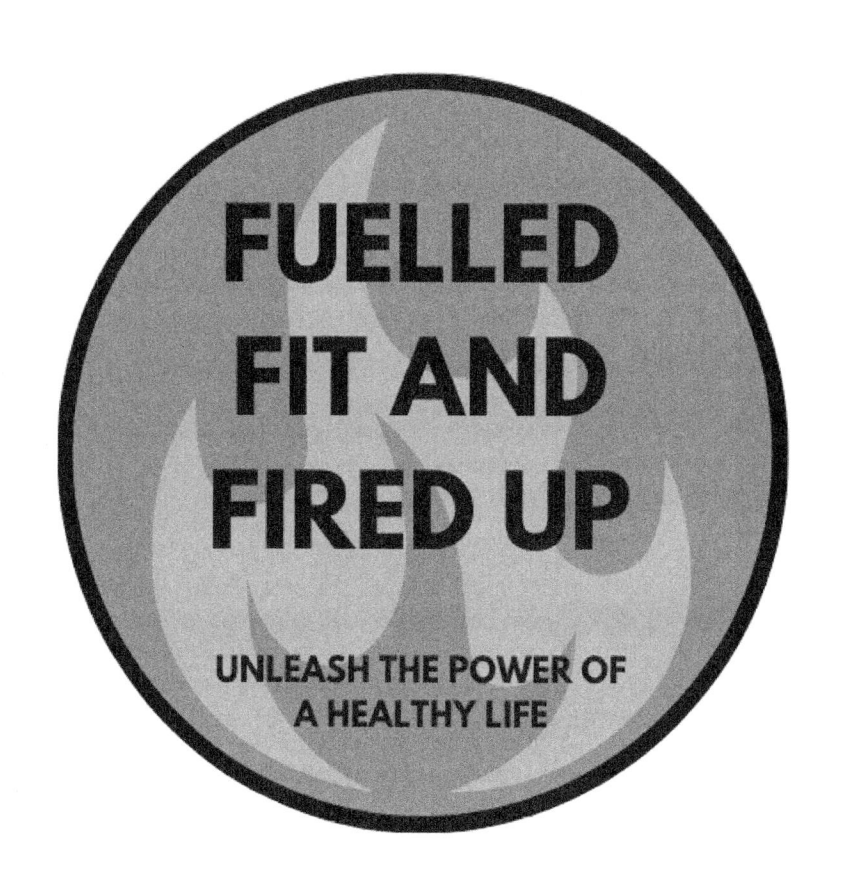

DAVID ROGERS
Foreword by Michael Heppell

FUELLED FIT AND FIRED UP
UNLEASH THE POWER OF A HEALTHY LIFE

Copyright © 2021 by David Rogers

All rights reserved. No part of this book may be reproduced or used in any manner without the author's written permission except for the use of quotations in a book review.

While the author has used their best efforts in preparing this book, they make no representations or warranties with respect to the accuracy or completeness of the contents of the book and specifically disclaims warranties of merchantability or fitness for a particular purpose.

This book's content is for information purposes only. There are no guarantees concerning the level of success you may experience by following the advice and strategies contained in this book. Please consult with your physician or a healthcare specialist regarding the suggestions and recommendations made, and you should take full responsibility for your safety and know your limits. Before trying any task, strategy, exercise, or recipe described in this book, be sure that your equipment is well maintained and do not take risks beyond your level of experience, aptitude, training, or comfort level. If you engage with any task, strategy, exercise, or recipe described in this book, you agree that you do so at your own risk. You are voluntarily participating in these activities, assume all risk of injury to yourself, and agree to release and discharge the author from all claims or causes of action, known or unknown, arising out of the contents of this book. The use of this book implies your acceptance of this disclaimer.

First Paperback Edition 2021
First E-Book Edition 2021
This edition 2021
ISBN 979-8-7122-3189-8
Independently Published via Kindle Direct Publishing

For my wife Amanda, and our three dogs
Thank you for all the fun, love, and support
Without it, I would never have finished this book

RIP Bertie
We will never forget you
Enjoy life at Rainbow Bridge
July 2009 - April 2020

TABLE OF CONTENTS

TABLE OF CONTENTS 7
FOREWORD BY MICHAEL HEPPELL 9
PREFACE 11
INTRODUCTION 15
1. YOU HAVE THE POWER 19
2. POWER YOUR FOUNDATIONS 27
3. POWER YOUR IMPOSTER 32
4. POWER YOUR HABITS 38
5. POWER YOUR MIND 48
6. POWER YOUR BREATHING 59
7. POWER YOUR SLEEP 68
8. POWER YOUR DETOX 75
9. POWER YOUR HYDRATION 91
10. POWER YOUR PLATE 97
11. POWER YOUR FITNESS 110
12. POWER YOUR PLANNING 129
13. POWER YOUR RESULTS 135
14. POWER YOUR PASSIONS 143
15. FINAL THOUGHTS 146
APPENDIX I: THE RECIPES 149
APPENDIX II: THE EXERCISES 187
ACKNOWLEDGMENTS 201
ABOUT THE AUTHOR 202
SOCIAL MEDIA 203

FOREWORD BY MICHAEL HEPPELL

If I could offer you a simple pill. A pill you take once, and that's it... you're done. The results are vigour, vitality, and vibrant health - forever. Who wouldn't take it? One pill, and you'll be feeling fantastic, sleeping well, waking with energy, looking in the mirror without breathing in, no aches or pains, and looking forward to a longer life.

As with any pill, there could be side effects. They include: starting to make better choices, moving more, and understanding how your body works. Feeling the urge to prepare delicious healthy meals, become super hydrated, and find more time to exercise. The pill doesn't make you a fanatic, but it does encourage you to test out new and interesting ideas and alternatives.

This pill isn't swallowed. But it is easily digested.

You're holding it.

Fuelled, Fit and Fired Up isn't a pill. It's better than that. Think of it as a guide to getting the very best out of life. There's a refreshing lack of complicated jargon and many nods to classic well-known ideas and concepts. The ones we know but don't necessarily do.

David Rogers is one of the kindest people I know. He joined my Facebook Group and quickly became our most active member. Every day David offers encouragement and support to other members and shares his ideas for a better, more enjoyable, healthier life.

He often posts a picture of a delicious meal he's created and quickly receives many comments. Mainly, 'Recipe please.' I was excited when he announced he was writing Fuelled, Fit and Fired Up and it would contain a recipe section too.

I love David's passion and couldn't wait to see it translated into a book. And here it is. Step by step, page by page, your guide to feeling Fuelled, Fit and Fired up every day.

Michael Heppell
Author, Coach, Speaker

PREFACE

The world is relentless. Every day throws up new, and not always, exciting challenges. Technology is taking over our lives, quenching our thirst for excitement through social media or the latest Netflix series. We have never been so time-poor, which is ironic given that life is much easier than for previous generations. The fact is the very things that make our lives more efficient are simply eating into our time even more.

How can we possibly find the time to eat healthier, get fitter, and feel amazing?

The million-dollar question?

Or a million-dollar excuse?

Putting up mental barriers is something we choose to do. We create a lie, a narrative. Convincing ourselves we can't change. Our perception of time prevents us from living a healthier lifestyle, and in the process, we miss out on the benefits it brings.

How do I know?

I was living that lie.

I was overweight, lacked energy, and I was nowhere near my best, physically or mentally. I didn't feel good, let alone great.

I was tired of being tired.

Things needed to change. I needed to change. I promised to improve my life and create a better future by being anchored in the present. Focused on the here and now, no longer worrying about the past or indeed what was to come. The goal was to eat healthier, get fitter, and focus on myself.

Making the promise was easy. How to deliver that promise was the challenge. To quote Mark Twain;

'Giving up smoking is the easiest thing in the world. I know because I've done it thousands of times.'

Taking that first step out of our comfort zone is hard. Staying out of it is even harder, as our fight or flight response tries to convince us to regress into bad habits.

We know new routines need time to form.

So, why do we give up so easily?

We don't like the pain that change brings. Our old ways provide comfort and assurance, and we actively seek out the pleasure associated with them.

The discipline of change is about breaking this cycle, and over time becoming comfortable with being uncomfortable. This evolution can provide happiness and energy in copious amounts. They are the rewards for creating a winning feeling, driven by our end goal of living a healthier life.

By setting ourselves three simple objectives, we can change our lives for the better.

1. Be Excited

2. Be Present

3. Be Curious

The first two relate to being in the present moment, aware of everything around us. The third is about rediscovering our childhood curiosity and opening our minds to new strategies, techniques, and ideas—all to create new habits that deliver sustainable lifestyle change.

The good news is you have already taken the difficult first step. You have recognised the need to change. Now you need to develop the how, inspired by a sense of purpose, driven by the reason you want to change. As you progress through this book, you will learn what you can do, how you can do it, and most importantly, why it works.

This book intends to help you unleash the power of a healthy life and reap the benefits in all aspects of it. It shares practical tips, techniques, and ideas, along with the knowledge I have gained along the way.

I hope you enjoy reading this book and that it helps you make that change.

INTRODUCTION

Healthy living will have a different meaning for everyone who reads this book. For some, it is what you eat. For others, it might be staying fit. In this book, you will find out there are several other ways to unleash the power of a healthy life.

This book is for *YOU*. To get the most out of it, consider how you interact with the content, engaging in a way that suits you. You could choose a flexible approach, flicking backward and forward between chapters, as each has its particular subject and learning. Equally, you may want to read the book from cover to cover. The choice is yours.

There may be chapters that you see as a must-read. Some you may not connect with immediately. Know that there is no right or wrong approach when it comes to reading this book. Ultimately, the changes you want to introduce are personal. Feeling comfortable with a process that delivers the best results for you is crucial.

The content combines challenging your belief system with how your brain recognises patterns and how you can ultimately form new habits. You can apply this knowledge to build a stable foundation that does not preclude you from having flexibility and adaptability in delivering your goals. The balance between these three attributes allows you to form new habits and, crucially, make them stick.

You will learn that rest and recovery are as equally important as what you consume. When it comes to health and fitness, the overall goal is to power both your physical and mental agility, providing the energy you need to make a difference in your life.

There will be subjects you enjoy, techniques you embrace, and ideas that stretch you. Perhaps some will make you feel self-conscious or uneasy. The purpose of sharing them is to challenge your current way of thinking, to deliver personal growth, and discover new healthier habits. They will help you become comfortable feeling uncomfortable. Accepting these feelings will make your experience even more enjoyable.

The ideas, information, and techniques help explain why previous attempts to change have perhaps not been as successful or permanent as you had hoped. You will find yourself empowered by the knowledge and having the ability to create new habits, delivering on your promise for a sustainable, healthier life.

To get the most out of the book, take time to consider the following.

BE HONEST

Take a good hard look at yourself in the mirror, which is never easy. Be truthful about the situation, accept the challenges that lie ahead, but always be kind to yourself. Remind yourself of why you want to change and the positive impact it will have on your life and potentially the lives of others. Honesty about why, what, and how you are going to change will only improve the results.

BE OPEN

Embrace the techniques, ideas, and suggestions. Take them on merit, and regularly apply what works for you. Nothing written in the book is a must-do. You can try everything or nothing. It's your effectiveness and willingness to implement it that delivers the change.

BE REFLECTIVE

Scribble in the margin, make notes in any blank spaces. Formulate your plans as you go, remembering to go back and reflect when you learn something new.

Each chapter ends with three questions that allow you to reflect on what you have read. They may be a What? How? Or When? And perhaps the occasional Who? All posed to help you think about the new habits that will improve your life. Why only three questions? Well, you will find that out in the next chapter.

Remember to be excited, be present, and most of all, be curious. Commit to learning something new, focus on the process, and step out of your comfort zone. The results will take care of themselves. And whether you embrace one or two techniques or apply everything to your life, you will change it for the better.

REFLECTION

Three, on the face of it, simple but perhaps challenging questions to begin.

1. **Why do you want to change?**

2. **What is your #1 goal to achieve?**

3. **Who else will benefit from these changes?**

1. YOU HAVE THE POWER

THE POWER OF THREE

The *Power of Three* will be a common theme throughout the book. It is the reason it's called Fuelled, Fit and Fired Up, a trifecta of alliteration to grab your attention and motivate change.

During childhood, the *Power of Three* captured your imagination without you even realising it. Progressing through this chapter will show you how influential it has been and how you can use it to inspire the changes you want to make.

The number three was important, inspiring, and influential on many parts of your early years' development. Your parents would sing *Three Blind Mice* to keep you entertained. Fantastic fairy tales were read to you at bedtime, including *Goldilocks and the Three Bears* and the *Three Little Pigs*. Both stories that have three characters provided three options. Walt Disney presented three good fairies in *Sleeping Beauty* and Donald Duck's nephews; *Huey, Louie, and Dewey*.

This pattern carried on into your education, with the three fundamental sciences being *Physics, Chemistry, and Biology*. Mathematics taught you about triangles and Pythagoras' Theorem, and the history books quote *Veni, Vidi, Vici – We Came, We Saw, We Conquered*.

As you move into adulthood, when anything untoward happens, you are reminded, *everything comes in threes*. You give *blood, sweat, and tears* to get that project over the line, and when choosing a new home, it is all about *location, location, location*.

It doesn't stop there, as advertisers and slogan writers love the *Power of Three*. *The Green Cross Code Man* taught you to *Stop, Look, and Listen*. *Nike* told you *Just Do It*, and you cannot beat the *Snap, Crackle, and Pop* of *Rice Krispies*.

The *Power of Three* is everywhere!

But why three?

Why not one or two?

Why is three the magic number? And how can it influence you again now?

Let's explore why in a little more detail. First up, good old number one. Signifying the first time, something special, but it is only ever at that specific moment. Your first words, first steps, or first attempt at driving are all fantastic achievements, but you can only have the first time, well, once. All the time, you are ticking tasks off your *to-do list* of life as you go.

Two is the binary number, signifying a choice between two options. Yes or No. Right or Wrong. Heads or Tails. That's all just a little bit boring.

But with three, that's when the magic happens. You can start creating basic patterns that engage your mind and body, enabling you to complete tasks, solve problems and form new habits. Let's delve into why this is the case.

NEUROSCIENCE AND PSYCHOLOGY

Your brain loves patterns, using them to solve problems, predict outcomes and learn new skills. You could say it is your very own internal *Power of Three*. So, it won't come as a surprise that the brain has three main parts.

Cerebrum (the front)
The most significant part, it's how you remember, problem solve, think, and feel.

Cerebellum (the back)
Under the cerebrum, just the back of the skull, this controls balance and coordination.

The Brain Stem (the middle)
Sitting beneath the cerebrum, in front of the cerebellum, this is the mother ship. It regulates the heart rate and, amongst other functions, your breathing, sleeping, and eating. It's one end of the information superhighway between the body and the brain.

The number three also influences your short-term memory, with it potentially challenging to remember lists of more than three items. How often have you been shopping without a list and forgotten several things? Or had to double-check a large drinks order at the coffee shop? Without applying specific techniques, it may be a regular occurrence.

But a list of three has distinct characteristics: *a start, a middle, and an end,* which provides natural rhythm when reciting it and making it more likely to be committed to memory. It is no coincidence that some of the best speechwriters use what they call *The Rule Of Three* when creating campaign slogans. Just take these three examples, Britain Deserves Better (UK Labour Party, 1997), Yes We Can (Barack Obama, 2008), or Strong and Stable (UK Conservative Party, 2017).

In Psychology, Abraham Maslow's motivational theory shows five levels to the hierarchical pyramid of needs. The human wants or desires that allow you to function at your best. In some more straightforward representations, there are only three levels; *basic, psychological, and self-fulfilment.*

Basic
These are physiological and safety needs, such as food, water, oxygen, and security.

Psychological
Need for love, belonging, and prestige, with an overarching feeling of accomplishment.

Self-Fulfilment
You achieve your potential through morality, creativity, and problem-solving.

In a 1967 speech, Dr. Martin Luther King Jr described it as the three dimensions of a complete life; *length, breadth, and height.*

Length
Searching out your inner power, learning to love yourself properly, and in his words, *'having the inward concern for one's welfare.'*

Breadth
You turn the view outward, focusing your concern on other people.

Height
This stage is where you seek out hope, meaning, or achievement.

Throughout this book, return to the *Power of Three* to help you focus and create new habits. New patterns that will deliver sustainable changes to your life. The next chapter explains how you can achieve balance through stability, flexibility, and adaptability. But, before you do that, you need to focus on the most important person.

AND THAT IS YOU.

Yes, YOU are the most important person.

By taking care of yourself first, you can unleash the power of a healthy life. You will operate in the upper levels of both Maslow's and Dr. King's hierarchies. A place where achieving outstanding results is a more regular occurrence.

Focusing on yourself first can be challenging. It's human nature to support, nurture and develop others. You experience both emotional and physical benefits when being kind and helpful, making you happier, giving a sense of purpose and meaning. Perhaps it even feels a little selfish to focus all your attention on yourself.

But without doing it, can you make that change?

Take a moment to reflect on how you spend your free time. How often are you recharging your batteries? Do you run around for others? While not focusing on you, your wellbeing is diminishing. By taking time for yourself, you are relaxing and rejuvenating the mind, body, and soul.

Putting it another way, if your mobile phone is at 10% charge, what action do you take? Typically, after a mild panic, you will recharge it. Nobody wants the battery, and phone, to run down entirely. So, why don't you apply the same logic to yourself? And recharge your battery before the red light starts flashing.

To achieve a peak state, physically, mentally, and emotionally, you must focus on yourself first. From a position of readiness and positivity, it becomes less challenging to negotiate the tsunami of life. Retraining this focus is not easy. You will have people who depend on you; *children, elderly relatives, or work colleagues*. You must take an uncharacteristic approach to life, fitting your face mask first, just as instructed during a flight safety briefing.

'If the cabin pressure changes suddenly during the flight, oxygen masks will automatically drop from the compartment above your seat. If this happens, pull one of the masks down to your face and cover your nose and mouth. ***Be sure to put your mask on before helping others*** *and keep it on until a crew member advises you to take it off.'*

How often during everyday life does your cabin pressure drop? And you find yourself in a challenging situation with others who may need support. In the briefing, you receive instructions to make sure you are safe before engaging in helping others. How often do you do this in real life?

By concentrating on your *state*, you will be able to impact and influence the situation, resolving any problems efficiently and effectively. There are three elements that can affect your *state*; *Physiology, Focus, and Language*.

Physiology

Known as the science of life, it refers to the interaction between your body, its interconnected systems, and the direct influences on them. How you breathe (chapter six), sleep (chapter seven), and nourish your body (chapters nine and 10) all impact physical, mental and emotional health.

Focus

By focusing on past events, any negative experiences can influence your results and success. By concentrating on the outcome, your mindset changes to one that allows you to achieve a peak state with increasing regularity. If your focus falters, use exercise (chapter 11) or meditation (chapter five) to centre the body, and remove any stress triggers.

Language

Sounds simple, but positive words drive positive behaviour. Your internal narrative influences your view of the world and how you allow it to impact you. Using positive language can change your emotional state. Removing words like don't, won't, can't, or but from your vocabulary is a great start. Next time you find yourself using negative language, stop, make a mental note and consider how you could have positively framed the sentence. As you slowly move towards more positive language, both your physiology and focus will change.

It is rare to operate at a peak state for a significant amount of time. But you can achieve it with increased regularity. By creating a positive mindset, you can control your emotion, reduce the negative influence of past experiences, and deliver positive outcomes. Don't be the person sitting at 10%, with your internal battery flashing. Plug yourself in and recharge.

Remember, you are the most important person, and you are in control of everything.

REFLECTION

In closing this chapter, let's focus on your *state*.

1. **What previous experiences do you allow to cloud your judgement, influence decision-making, or stop you from acting?**

2. **How do you feel about how these affect your life?**

3. **How can you introduce more positive language into your vocabulary?**

2. POWER YOUR FOUNDATIONS

At the time of writing, the Burj Khalifa is the world's tallest building. Standing at the height of 830 metres and weighing in at 500,000 tonnes, it soars majestically above the glittering metropolis of Dubai. Solid and stable foundations are the order of the day to hold that behemoth in a freestanding form. But it is what happens when the winds race across the desert that is interesting.

Not unlike other modern skyscrapers, the Burj Khalifa can sway in the wind. The building is tuned like a musical instrument, so the internal harmonics don't coincide with the wind's rhythmic nature. The sway of the building is slow, to not affect anyone visiting or living in the structure. The building has become flexible and adaptable to the external environment while keeping its core stability—a fantastic set of characteristics to possess.

Consider how you could soar to peak performance by adopting stability, flexibility, and adaptability as your core characteristics.

Real life is a little more complicated than just dealing with the wind though. Stimuli come continuously and simultaneously from various sources, quickly knocking you off course if you let them. Social media can sensationalise the smallest of issues, amplifying negativity and trigger a crisis response. And in this instance, it's not just global or national events causing the worry.

You face personal challenges daily, all potentially impacting your life more than any worldwide event. You may have lost a loved one, struggled with mental health, or suffered the breakdown of a relationship. Regardless of the event, one thing remains consistent. You feel a complete loss of control, as external influences have affected your *state* and amplified your reaction to the situation.

Those with a cool head make informed, rational decisions. They operate at a *peak state* more regularly, in complete control of their physiology, focus, and language. You could describe it as personal stability, having firm foundations on which a successful and healthier life will flourish. It affords you the energy to address any challenge, with you thinking and acting clearly, remaining flexible and adaptable to the situation. You may even find solutions to problems that you didn't know you had.

How can you create this stability? Well, it is perhaps more straightforward than you think.

In the previous chapter, you read about the *Power of Three*, how it influences your life, and at times without you realising. Stability, with flexibility and adaptability, can become your *Power of Three*. To understand why and how, consider this question.

Why do photographers use a tripod?

Because it guarantees balance, there is stability, reducing the risk of blurry images in the photographs. It is their *Power of Three*, a real-world application of Mathematics and Physics. Three contact points creating an even triangular plane, regardless of how uneven the floor or the length of the tripod's legs. The photographer has a stable base, flexible and adaptable to the environment around it. Simple adjustments can level the camera with ease, just as straightforward techniques can help you change.

Apply this logic to your life, with each leg of the proverbial tripod representing a positive influence that can impact your physical, mental, or emotional health. The renewed vigour gives you the power to handle everything that life throws at you, subconsciously preparing you for things before they happen. You have stability, flexibility, and adaptability through a triangular plane of wellbeing, aligned with Maslow's hierarchy of needs or Dr. King's dimensions of life (refer back to chapter one if you need a reminder).

By improving how you fuel your body and keep it fit, you get fired up and unleash the power of a healthy life. Let's take a look at Fuelled, Fit and Fired Up in a little more detail.

FUELLED

Do you consider yourself as someone who lives life on the edge?

Perhaps you play chicken with the fuel gauge on your car. An exciting prospect until you lose, and your vehicle and life grind to a halt. But even if you have a full tank, it has to be the correct fuel. Diesel in a petrol engine, or visa versa, is never a good combination. Yes, you might get a few miles out of it, but the outcome is catastrophic and costly.

Your body is no different. With the wrong fuel, you don't perform at your best in many areas of life. By introducing minor changes to the food and drink consumed, you can ensure energy levels are improved, and you operate effectively and efficiently. But it's not just about what you eat and drink. How you fuel your body through sleep, the way your breath, and how to clear your mind and body of toxins can all improve your health.

FIT

At some point in your life, you will have promised yourself to get fit or at least fitter. You may have signed up for that gym membership in January, *'new year new me'* you will have said to yourself. And then May rolls around, and you've been twice. Both life and time have got away from you.

At this point, it is worth reminding yourself that recognising you want to change is the first and hardest step. Approaching each subsequent phase becomes more straightforward as you apply the techniques and ideas, learn how to form new habits, maintain the momentum, and ultimately improve your fitness.

FIRED UP

Everyone has different passions. Those pastimes and hobbies they enjoy or new skills and knowledge they want to learn. You are no different. Being at the peak of your power, through health and fitness, will make growing your mind that much easier. With more energy comes better learning. The world becomes your oyster when it comes to personal development. You can arm yourself with the knowledge that not only helps others but helps you deal with real-life situations. Applying simple but effective techniques allows you to thrive in your passions.

REFLECTION

Buildings need to have stable foundations and are never built on quicksand as they would rapidly sink.

1. What stops you from developing your foundations for life, dragging you into the proverbial quicksand in the process?

2. How can improving your health and fitness help address these issues?

3. How do you currently feel about your chances of success?

3. POWER YOUR IMPOSTER

Have you ever felt like a fraud? That you don't deserve success or happiness? Or that at any moment, family, friends, or work colleagues might find you out?

The good news is that if this is you, you are not alone. Most people have had these feelings at one time or another. It's one of the biggest challenges you face when approaching change and trying to achieve extraordinary results. It is more commonly known as:

IMPOSTER SYNDROME

Even if you haven't heard of it, you will have experienced imposter syndrome at some point in your life. That nagging doubt, manifesting itself as a lack of confidence, stopping you from growing and succeeding. Around 70% of people admit to having that little devil sitting on their shoulder, providing them with all the reasons not to act. You might be one of those people, but don't worry if you are because you are in great company. There are many famous people, admired for successful careers, who have suffered from it.

US actor Tom Hanks has spoken in interviews about thinking about being viewed as a fraud. He is perhaps questioning his success, worried about being discovered as a fake. All this from a man who has not one but two Best Actor Oscars sitting on his mantlepiece.

Sheryl Sandberg, the Chief Operating Officer of Facebook, talks about believing she had fooled everyone, every time she didn't embarrass herself or even when she excelled. In her words, she was worried that *'one day soon, the jig would be up.'*

And the final celebrity *'imposter'* is nine-time Grammy Award winning musician Lady Gaga. She has spoken about still feeling like a loser from high school, despite multi-million record sales and worldwide success. She reminds herself every morning that she is a superstar to help her get through the day.

You are not alone in these obstructive thoughts, but they can create feelings of anxiety, stress, or guilt. Which then manifest in negative responses to challenge and change. Why does that have to be the case? And how can you flip it on its head?

The ability to recognise Imposter Syndrome is key to delivering change and those fantastic results you crave. By acknowledging its existence, you can prepare for its appearance and even embrace it as a driver of change. Every time you face a new challenge, it's natural to be fearful, worried, or uneasy about the situation. It's part of the learning process, and the first thing to be aware of is that you react in one of two ways. In both cases, delaying positive action, but they are polar opposite approaches.

Procrastination

You delay the task, that little devil telling you that you can't do it, won't do it, or just don't want the hassle. Finding any excuse to postpone the challenge, avoiding pain rather than embracing the pleasure the result brings.

Over Preparation

You leave no stone unturned, seeking the perfect outcome, delaying final action until you are 100% happy.

The bad news is you will never achieve this utopia, as perfection doesn't exist.

But there is good news. In striving for perfection, you can achieve excellence, but only if you take immediate positive action. With no effort too small, all progress is good progress. The best and most sustainable results come from continuous improvement through marginal gains across several different areas. The Japanese have a term for it, *Kaizen*, meaning *'change for the better.'* Invented by Masaaki Imai, many companies successfully and consistently use it to deliver improvement and change. The car manufacturer Toyota is one of the most recognisable proponents of Kaizen.

Sports teams are now embracing marginal gains, with the hugely successful British and Sky cycling teams implementing the philosophy, as they won race after race. They say success breeds success, and you only have to look at dominating dynasties across all sports to find the evidence. You can apply this formula with equal success, accepting the feelings of imposter syndrome and turning them to your advantage.

Take another look at the three incredibly successful individuals mentioned earlier in this section. All at the top of their industries, but all suffering doubts. Does this suggest success increases imposter syndrome? Maybe it does, but what Tom, Sheryl, and Gaga have in common is that they have overcome those feelings, and you can too.

By taking a positive view of imposter syndrome, you can embrace the devil whispering in your ear and allow it to empower you.

POSITIVES OF IMPOSTER SYNDROME

You Recognise That You Are Challenging Yourself

You want to push yourself, move out of your comfort zone, and make those lifestyle changes. It may feel awkward, perhaps even painful, but you must challenge any societal and personal norms to grow. By recognising and embracing this feeling, you know you are making progress, moving positively toward your end goal.

Leaves Your Ego At The Door

There is a fine line between confidence, fashioned from self-belief, and arrogance, manifesting from perceived superiority. But the step between arrogance and stupidity is even smaller. When your ego takes over, you fail to observe potential unknowns, leading to mistakes or failure. Imposter syndrome grounds you, makes you think about your actions, and focuses on the achievements. Harness the positive feelings from both the route you have taken and outcomes along the way.

It's A Sign Of Growth

As you become accomplished, your knowledge increases, and you feel a sense of achievement. At this moment, imposter syndrome arises, and those doubts start flying around. That devil on your shoulder tells you that *'you don't deserve this success.'* By acknowledging this trigger, you can embrace the feelings for what they are, positive affirmations that what you are doing is working. You can start celebrating the wins rather than wallowing in doubt.

HOW TO TURN IT INTO A POSITIVE

Find A Support System

Surround yourself with a trusted inner circle, those sources of encouragement, such as family, friends, or a group of like-minded people. You will know who they are, people that say just the right thing, at just the right moment. They may even recognise when you are falling into the clutches of imposter syndrome before you even realise it. Some people may call it an accountability group, and there is more about them in chapter 13.

You can use this network to help find simple ways to reminisce about previous successes, share recognition, or provide a simple well done. It will serve you well, and you can wheel out these positive feelings when that little devil appears.

You Are Your Own Person

Online platforms create constant comparisons and a drive for social acceptance. Neither are healthy obsessions, and it becomes easy to get caught up in it all. Nobody is perfect, so you don't have to be. You are an individual, so embrace imperfection, trust your process, and deliver what you can control.

Fill Your Head With Positive Thoughts

Think more positively. Sounds easy but is often challenging. With self-doubt always there, negative thoughts become established based on previous experience. If you accept them as historical events, you can tune out from what has happened before. Mindfulness (chapter five) helps focus on the present moment, allowing you to concentrate on how you feel and your current success. By celebrating these wins, you will continue to move forward, building a bank of positive thoughts as you go. Sometimes you have just got to remind yourself of the value you bring to your life.

Life is unpredictable, challenging, and at times relentless. You are often moving at a hundred miles an hour, struggling to keep up with life, let alone getting fired up about it. It creates an environment where imposter syndrome can thrive. By taking a step back, you can swap the negative for positive, embrace the feelings imposter syndrome brings, and permit yourself to keep moving forward. You can slay your fears and anxiety in the process.

The magic happens outside your comfort zone. Sow the seeds and watch them bloom.

REFLECTION

Think of a situation where you experienced a feeling of self-doubt or were worried about '*being found out.*'

1. **How did you react?**

2. **What could you have done differently to recognise the positivity in the situation?**

3. **When you try something new, who provides the most encouragement?**

4. POWER YOUR HABITS

You know you want to change, but perhaps not understanding what or how makes it challenging. In the first few chapters, you have reflected on several questions. You now know why you want to change, some of the barriers that are stopping you, and that you must react positively to any challenges

Now it is time to start looking at techniques that will help you form new habits—allowing you to take that first step out of your comfort zone. It is essential to recognise that in developing new habits and routines, you will make mistakes. Learn to embrace them, taking time to observe the imperfection. Become comfortable with it. After all, a flawed diamond is worth more than a perfect pebble.

Throughout this chapter, you will learn about possible reactions you need to address, abilities to develop or rediscover, and the habit loop.

BREAKING PROMISES

Having made the promise to change, you can often fail to commit. Creating a narrative to convince yourself it is acceptable not to act. This failure to engage stops the contract you made with yourself from being upheld. Your dreams will stay as dreams if you don't commit.

Your brain creates patterns that determine behaviour, in turn influencing your internal belief system. Your inner narrative is convincing you that decisions are for the better when the reality is that you are avoiding pain. It is a protective response, known as *fight or flight*. Particular events or situations activate your stress response, which in turn clouds your decision-making capability, and you settle on keeping yourself safe.

If you notice these internal lies, stop building the evidence to justify the poor decision. As the untruths present themselves, take the opportunity to turn them into a positive outcome and take action rather than avoiding it. Simply put, stop making excuses.

By reflecting on this notion, sometimes known as *false will*, you can explore specific influences, ideas, and techniques to deliver on your promise to change.

BOUNCEBACKABILITY

You may know it better as resilience, the way to recover from or adjust easily to misfortune or change. An ability you have as a child but seemingly forget as adulthood takes control. Take some time to reflect on how you learnt to ride a bike. If that's too long ago, remind yourself what happened when you taught the kids.

When they tipped sideways from their bike and crashed to the floor, what happened next? In most cases, up they bounce, and after a few tears, they are ready to try again. As you move into adulthood, a more risk-averse approach to these types of failure takes over. Perhaps it is a better understanding of the situation, but worry about worst-case scenarios often becomes the norm.

Dwelling on the pain, suffering, or negativity a decision causes will not breed change. Embrace your inner child, and don't be scared of making the wrong choice. Accept that, on the odd occasion, you may *fall off your bike*. It is how you react in returning to these bad experiences with health and fitness that is important. Recognise the imperfection, focus on your desired results, and move back toward positive association with the change.

Hosting a pity party, perhaps where you comfort eat to block out negative influences, only helps in the short term. Wallowing is fine, but don't get stuck in the mud. Pick yourself up, dust yourself down and keep moving forward. Just like you did as a child.

CURIOSITY

When did you last learn something new? A skill or a subject that was alien to you. Have you ever considered changing careers? Most people don't because they're comfortable and are concerned about not knowing what they don't know.

Curiosity was an essential ingredient of your childhood. Your parents faced a barrage of questions as you tried to learn about this big wide world. They were continually met with, Why? When? What? and How? You grew knowledge, learnt skills, and developed behaviours, blissfully ignorant of certain situations.

To inspire that curiosity and a feeling of achievement, toys such as Lego may have been commonplace in your early years. You would paint, draw and explore. Perhaps you took toys apart to find out how they worked. All in the name of curiosity. It is no coincidence that adults re-engage with Lego later in life. Child-like curiosity has resurfaced.

As you grow older, negative experiences or societal norms start censoring this curiosity. The risk of embarrassment stops us from asking stupid questions, preventing further growth. Nobody wants to put their head above the parapet, only to get shot down. The risk of adverse or negative reactions and comments on social media breeds the same feeling. Why put yourself in that situation?

Those that continue to develop, who facilitate change in their lives, don't care what people think. A sage piece of advice. Why? Because it is how you feel and act upon the promised change that is most important.

By accepting new habits that initially feel uncomfortable, you can change things for the better. Embrace *every day as a school day*, regardless of your age and experience.

THE HABIT LOOP

There are numerous approaches to creating or changing habits. The length of time or number of repetitions needed varies with individuals. The key lies in the habit loop, made up of three distinct parts; *the cue, the routine, and the reward*. As you form new habits, the circle is broken and then rebuilt with better decisions.

When choosing the habit you want to break, first, make the cue invisible. Next, force the routine to be complicated or unattractive, then the reward becomes unsatisfying. Flipping the logic creates a new habit. An obvious cue, with an easy, attractive routine, naturally develops a satisfying reward.

To illustrate this point, consider this scenario.

Your morning alarm sounds, you feel a bit tired, and the snooze button becomes your new best friend. An everyday occurrence. Another hour in bed. Amazing!

Do you get up feeling amazing?
Do you feel rewarded?
Probably not.

The reality is you end up scrambling around getting ready for work, rushing to grab everything to get the kids to school, and your work commute turns into a disaster. You miss your usual train or rush hour traffic derails your journey. Life is not going to plan.

Now let's take a different view, breaking the situation into the three constituent parts of the habit loop. You will see it's easier to form a new habit than you think.

The Cue

The alarm is sounding, and that triggers the start of the habit. Do you change the time? You could, but to what end. Making it earlier reduces the time you are sleeping. You are already tired when you wake. Depriving yourself of further shut-eye isn't going to help, as you will see in chapter 7 (Power Your Sleep).

The Routine

A simple change here. You get up and start the day as you mean to go on, take control, and attack your tasks. Grab some water to kick start your metabolism, and the energy soon starts to flow.

The Reward(s)

There is no rushing around by taking straightforward action, resulting in less stress and a better mood. You could use the additional time to instil a new habit, perhaps cook a healthier breakfast or take exercise. Both provide energy to fire you up for the day ahead.

Just one simple change has turned the situation on its head. Taking positive action has created attractive rewards, with this new outcome having the potential to develop compounded benefits as you embed your new habit.

BEAT THE WEEK

An excellent method for changing eating habits or building regular fitness plans, this steady and methodical approach delivers long-lasting change. It is comfortable, rewarding, and embraces imperfection.

Beat the Week is built on the principle of moderation and delivering consistent results. The underlying rule being you have more good days than bad. You may exercise four days out of seven or eat healthily for five days. The technique allows you to build slowly towards your desired outcomes.

In chapter one, you read that the language you use is crucial. Let's put this into practice. Perhaps you want to reduce unhealthy snacks in your diet, but eat crisps or chocolate every day. You enjoy them, but deep down, know they are not healthy. How do you approach it? What language do you use? You may use the words *'I need to STOP eating crisps.'* But you are defining an end, and this may feel uncomfortable.

What if you change your language and say the following instead, *'I want to REDUCE the number of crisps I'm eating?'* A slightly different approach, recognising the adverse impact on your health but permitting yourself to eat them.

By taking a systematic approach, you can make the change sustainable. In the first week, replace crisps with fruit on Monday. A subtle difference, but it sows the seed of change. The following week try the same on two days, increasing by a day every week. Within a month, you are beating the week, eating healthier, and have possibly realised you didn't like crisps as much as you thought.

By applying this technique to your weekly meal plan, you can steadily increase the number of healthy meals you are eating. Consider introducing a reward system, collecting gold stars for every healthy meal consumed. Once you have ten, allow yourself a treat of your choosing. With 21 mealtimes a week, you can have two treats if you work hard at being healthy.

VISUALISATION

Visualisation is a practice of changing thoughts, using your imagination to develop new habits. You create positive outcomes, using multi-sensory patterns to experience new behaviours and activities. You are creating new sequences in your mind, templates that your brain will recognise and associate with delivering successful results. It is a great technique to help achieve your goals and is easier to adopt than you think.

How often do you reminisce about a fantastic holiday or trip? Or a place you have worked? Even being at school, and the fun you have with friends? These are all visualisations. You are reminding yourself of brilliant times, the experience, the feelings, and the stimuli.

Elite athletes, such as Muhammad Ali, the self-professed greatest, use visualisation. Before every fight, he famously created his *Future History*. Over the weeks and days leading up to a fight, Ali would picture the end of the battle, his arms aloft, the referee proclaiming him the winner.

These visions became so vivid, and the unrelenting belief he would be successful became the norm. He imagined the crowds clapping and cheering, shouting his name, and the fantastic feeling of victory.

He was in the zone, all his energy and focus directed to make it happen. As he entered the ring, he was both mentally and physically prepared, having already won the fight in his mind. Subconsciously, he was constantly looking for ways to win and make the desired outcome a reality.

Modern elite athletes are no different, generating a vision of positive outcomes in an event or training session. Whether scoring a goal, hitting a home run, or lifting the trophy, they fashion each step to success in their mind. They even use it to relax and unwind, creating a calm environment to help maximise results. Being able to step into those feelings at any given time can create desired outcomes and personal best performances.

And you can use it too!

By imagining the details of success, thinking about how it looks, how you feel, and how it sounds, you include visual, kinaesthetic, and auditory learning. You are rehearsing the process, enhancing skills through repetition just as you would with physical practice. It is so powerful, being able to call on those images at any given time, training your mind and body to deliver your desired outcomes. It could be healthier eating, completing that run, or securing that new job. The technique is universal, applicable to any challenge, and you may even be using it without realising and achieving great results!

If visualisation is new to you, then here is how you start. First, embrace the power of your mind to create new ways of thinking and the ability to recognise patterns. In the beginning, this may feel uncomfortable or unnatural. To make it easier, try thinking about daily activities, perhaps climbing the stairs. Think about how it makes your body feel. Your heart may be racing, your breathing heavier than usual, or you might take it all in your stride. Whatever your thoughts, feelings, or visions, it shows you the power of your imagination.

These are some additional techniques to help you start your visualisation journey. Try them all and see what works for you.

Reminiscence

A simple technique that can kick-start changing your neural pathways and retrain your brain to form new habits. Close your eyes and begin remembering journeys to your favourite place. Remind yourself of the landmarks, the sounds, smells, and positive feelings you had. In your mind, revisit this place often, notice new things, which enhances your neurological pathways. Develop the ability to retrieve these thoughts whenever you need them.

Self-Talk

Take careful consideration of the language you use. Don't put undue pressure on yourself by being too demanding. Avoid using should, must, and have, moving your internal dialogue to preferences, such as want. Your desire for action increases, and success becomes more likely. You are talking yourself into positive results.

Repetition, Repetition, Repetition

New habits are formed by repeating new techniques, which extinguish those previous unhelpful behaviours. Regularly practicing visualisation will create new templates in your mind, easily accessible through memories.

Start Short Term

Take five minutes out of your day to practise goal visualisation. Imagine the steps that deliver your goal, making visions as authentic as possible. Including when, where, and who makes them more vivid.

Familiarity

Images of familiar objects help cement new feelings and thoughts. Things that you regularly encounter during your progress remind you of the journey and goal. You can think about buildings that you may pass while exercising, the fresh food aisle at the supermarket, or that soft pillow to improve your sleeping pattern. Make the visualisation as specific as possible to your goal.

Process And Outcome

To make your change sustainable, focus on what you want to achieve (the outcome) and how you will deliver it (the process). Visualise the steps along the way as well as the final goal. This intense focus will make the change more effective and long-lasting.

Remember that developing new healthier habits take time. Combining these techniques with recognising how and understanding why you sabotage your results can make your changes more sustainable.

REFLECTION

Forming new habits is the cornerstone to making changes to your life. But to do something new, you have to stop something else.

1. What bad habits do you want to break?
2. How are you going to approach it?
3. What will success look like for you?

5. POWER YOUR MIND

Your brain is a supercomputer that relays messages backward and forward, rapidly processing information through your senses. It allows you to think, experience, and create, the core of human intelligence.

For it to remain a highly effective and efficient machine, it has to be protected and maintained. And just as technological performance slows if a computer reaches capacity or software is not updated, your internal processor, the brain, reacts in the same way.

A relentless flow of information, 24 hours a day, seven days a week, continuously stimulates your senses. As your brain becomes crowded, it becomes increasingly difficult to make clear and conscious decisions. To truly unleash the power of your new healthier lifestyle, you must be able to make rational choices. As with a hard drive, taking time to defragment and organise the information you hold improves your effectiveness and efficiency. You should only retain what is essential and valuable, ensuring you operate at peak state more regularly. Thus, allowing you to concentrate on creating an environment that will enable you to flourish.

At this point, it is worth remembering that you won't get it 100% right, 100% of the time. Nobody does. It is all about setting yourself up for consistent success, creating the time and space to enable a new mindset to blossom. Don't worry, because excellent results will not be far behind.

To help you find this headspace, you will now explore three techniques; *Mindfulness, Meditation, and the Mind*

Dump. They are all aimed at facilitating considered, structured, and correct decision-making. Strategies to clear the mind of irrelevant information, to focus on the outcomes, and designed to give you the capacity to think effectively. You are making your internal hard drive more stable, allowing suitable decisions to be made more regularly.

The three techniques won't provide a quick fix, but being flexible and adaptable to them all could give you the best results. You may try them and think '*no, not for me thanks,*' or home in on one that fits your circumstances best. There is one thing for sure. You will never know without attempting them.

MINDFULNESS

'a mental state achieved by focusing one's awareness on the present moment, while calmly acknowledging and accepting one's feelings, thoughts, and bodily sensations.'

How often do you give time and attention to what is happening in the moment? Consciously, taking a break from the world, removing all past and future feelings that trigger your emotional and behavioural responses. The practice of mindfulness reconnects you with the sensations that your body experiences at that moment. Practising it can help you understand yourself, your reactions, and what triggers them. You will become able to enjoy life to the maximum, more often.

Next time you are out for a walk in the countryside, take time to enjoy that moment, absorb the sensory stimuli, and experience a new view of the world. It could be the sound of the birds, the wind brushing your face, or watching a squirrel bound across the branches. They are all things you may typically take for granted.

Consider each of your five senses; sight, taste, touch, hearing, and smell. How often do you focus on them at that precise moment, how they make you feel, and how are they impact and influence your response to your environment?

Mindfulness increases this awareness, helping to improve your mental wellbeing by focusing on the present. You remove thoughts of the past and worries for the future, allowing your brain to identify patterns in your feelings and decision-making. Perhaps even highlighting the triggers of stress or anxiety, enabling you to take stock, reflect, and recognise these events.

By understanding this, you can create different, more positive outcomes and viewpoints to any challenge. You are training your brain to focus on the here and now, removing these prior or future events that can cloud judgement. This increased positivity allows you to combat the negative feelings of stress and anxiety, both linked with an increased risk of depression.

To help become comfortable with mindfulness, follow these three simple ideas.

Set Aside Formal Practice Time

When you first start mindfulness, choose the same time of day to practice. Perhaps your morning journey to work, straight after a gym session or while on your lunch break. To avoid distraction, create a quiet space, away from the humdrum of life. You can sit silently and focus on your thoughts, the sounds, and how you breathe. Follow the sensations through your body. You are always bringing your attention back to the present moment, and formal practice makes applying the technique more comfortable in daily life.

Practice Regularly

It is easy to allow your mind to run away. Autopilot takes over, and you start to focus on a bad experience or worry about an event yet to come. Through regular practice, you learn how to bring yourself back to the present moment, taking back control of your thoughts, feelings, and sensations.

Practice Different Approaches

As you become more comfortable with mindfulness, you can start varying when and where you practise. Whatever time of day it is, sit and allow yourself to become aware of the world around you. Concentrate on the feelings and sensations it creates, always bringing yourself back to that moment if your mind wanders. A different seat on the train or another chair in the office may give you a different perspective on how you feel. By varying these sensations, you become more comfortable accepting the feelings and start to view the world differently.

If you find you are struggling to focus, consider trying this technique to distance yourself from those negative thoughts running through your mind.

The Mind Bus

Imagine you are the driver of a bus full of passengers. Assign each thought about a specific negative experience or habit to a different person, giving each a unique voice and personality. These thoughts and feelings could be about unhealthy eating, the stress caused by a lack of sleep, or even finding the time to exercise. Choose something that will make your life better in the long term.

In your mind, apply different techniques to take control of the bus. You may visualise passengers leaving the bus or instructing them that you, as the driver, are in charge. As you follow this process, your thoughts become less potent. You see the passengers, or your thoughts, for what they are, temporary experiences passing through your life.

MEDITATION

Where mindfulness is about thinking in the present, meditation performs the factory reset, attempting to clear the mind completely. The technique creates an environment of relaxation that, amongst other benefits, allows you to stay calm throughout the day.

You may have a preconception about meditation. That it is sitting cross-legged, under a tree, burning incense while chanting *'Ohm.'* There is much more to it than that, and while mantras can be a large part of the process, this is not the only method to afford you the satisfaction meditation brings. Later in this section, you will learn practical, everyday approaches for you to try. But be warned, one does involve chanting.

Before all of that, let's explore the benefits of meditation in more detail.

BENEFITS OF MEDITATION

Reduced Anxiety

Your *fight or flight* reaction is triggered by the *amygdala,* the part of the brain that controls emotional and behavioural responses. It fires pulses along our neural pathways, travelling to another section of the brain called the *medial prefrontal cortex.* This is your assessment centre, the part of the brain used for decision making. It is here where you determine whether the *amygdala* alarm is justified or not.

By practising meditation, you can rewire this function, breaking down the current neural pathways. As you reduce the *flight* sensations, you start building new stronger neural links to the assessment centre. In turn creating more reasoned and rational responses, making you less likely to react with an explosion of emotion. With only 20 minutes of meditation, you will see significant reductions in your anxiety and agitation.

Improved Creativity

By practising techniques where you are aware of your feelings, thoughts, or sensations, you can improve creative thinking. These are known as open monitoring meditations and help enhance divergent thinking when attempting to solve complex problems.

Improved Memory

Meditation removes distraction and increases productivity, a combination that can improve rapid memory recall. Being able to remind yourself quickly of positive outcomes will be essential to creating your new habits.

At first, meditation might feel daunting, a little unusual, and maybe even uncomfortable. After all, you don't have much time to sit and reflect on your innermost thoughts. It is essentially doing nothing, a task your brain actively avoids. But don't be concerned, as you are not alone in these feelings. Over thousands of years, there are millions of people who felt the same before their first practice.

Meditation will give you a better perspective on life, which can change dramatically the more you practice. Apply different techniques to produce different outcomes, finding out what works best. You want an approach that gives you the essence of feeling at one with your world.

For those that are new to meditation, here are some techniques to get you started.

Breathing Meditations

These focus on the process and feelings associated with breathing, freeing your mind of all past, present, and future thoughts. Start sitting upright in a chair, close your eyes, keep your feet planted to the ground, and have your hands resting loosely on your lap or knees. Place your attention on how your body feels while breathing, focusing on your chest and abdominal movement as they rise and fall.

Focus Meditations

Choose an object, such as a flower or candle, to form the focus of these meditations. Zero in on the object's details, the look, smell, and feel, all stimulating your senses to create a feeling of relaxation.

Walking Meditations

Derived from Zen Buddhist's meditation practices, these involve walking in silence, observing the world around you, taking in all the sounds, sights, and smells. If you find it challenging sitting in silence without distraction, then this style of practice will help.

Progressive Muscle Relaxation Meditations

Perhaps the simplest form of meditation, you contract and relax muscles throughout the body. By creating a flow from the top of your head to the bottom of your feet, you slowly move through the major muscle groups. It is both soothing and relaxing, and being a straightforward technique, it is excellent for beginners.

Mantra Meditations

Mantras are simple sounds or words repeated either silently or aloud. Based on the age-old practice of chanting, this technique provides you with focus and clarity. Many traditional mantras, such as *Om*, *Elohim*, or *So Ham*, are simple to learn. Finding a word or phrase related to your health goals can improve results.

There is no good or bad meditation practice, with your level of awareness being the measure of success. With no guarantee for a lifetime of happiness or solutions to all your problems, meditation will change the way you think, feel, and react to the challenges around you. The environment you create is one of relative calmness against a backdrop of chaos going on around you, just like the calm at the eye of a storm.

Any changes you experience through meditation will be gradual, as you slowly see and feel growing awareness of how you think about yourself and others. By practising regularly, the openness to challenge and willingness to change increases over time.

As with mindfulness, it is vital to find a rhythm and regularity, perhaps practising at the same time each day. You could pair it with another activity, known as *habit stacking*, so you always remember to meditate. Early in the morning is a great time to create a new habit, but you know your daily routine and where and when it will work for you.

Regularly remind yourself why you want to meditate and what goals you want to achieve. It will strengthen your commitment to take action, increase motivation, and build momentum.

MIND DUMP

As you read at the beginning of the chapter, your brain needs maintenance like any other piece of machinery. Processing a constant barrage of information reduces your version of bandwidth, with the ability to make decisions becoming less effective and less efficient. Consequently, your mental capacity to cope with situations or challenges reduces, and your energy levels wane. You slow down, just like broadband does with an increasing number of devices drawing from it. It is essential to clear space, creating the capacity to address challenges with a rational mind.

While mindfulness and meditation are techniques that people have adopted for thousands of years, the concept of mind dumping is a more modern approach to clearing thoughts or feelings from your head. Decluttering your mind in this way allows you to become creative about the task at hand. Many authors use the technique, with it facilitating creative writing and expressive thoughts about their ideas.

Applying this simple technique can help you focus on the essential changes you want to introduce. And the three steps couldn't be more straightforward. Now, grab a piece of paper, a pen and give it a go.

Step One

Write down everything that comes into your head. Yes, literally everything. Free flow, and don't worry about editing, spelling, or grammar. Don't stop. No thinking. Just dump your thoughts.

Step Two

Once you have exhausted your thoughts, feelings, and ideas, put your ramblings to one side. Take a moment, close your eyes and take three deep breaths. You could try the 3-

4-5 technique, which is in the next chapter (Power Your Breathing).

Step Three

Now go back to your list, exploring each random note further, and start answering the following questions. What do you need to expand upon? What are you thinking about right now? What is the next decision you need to take? And finally, how can your mind dump provide the answer? Challenge yourself by answering the questions that someone might ask if they found your ramblings. Take the time to cleanse your mind of all fears, anxieties, and stress.

Now you have done that, what's next?

You can start categorising your tasks, thoughts, or feelings, beginning to secure solutions in the process. Consider what is important or urgent, and remove those trivial tasks or problems, freeing yourself of worry and gaining time to address the most pressing issues.

This process of writing your thoughts down, creating a reference point, and the associated solutions is hugely important. Don't think about anything on the list until action is required. Instead, use the headspace to focus on your immediate challenges, and more rational and effective responses will flow.

The mind dump is a fantastic technique if you need to relax or are struggling with sleep. Practice before you go to bed, clearing your head of everything racing around from your daily activities. You can also keep a notepad and pen by your bed, then if you wake up with your mind racing, dump those thoughts straight away before drifting back to sleep.

Adopting any or all of the techniques in this chapter will help clear your mind and produce new and innovative solutions to your problems. Ultimately, you will be more effective at addressing any issues.

QUICK WIN

If you are not sure about the three main techniques shared in the chapter, try reducing your phone time and turn off your notifications. Social and traditional media channels provide written, visual and aural stimuli 24 hours, seven days a week. It is easy to become overwhelmed. Taking the news once a day, or reducing social media interaction, helps avoid wasted time and filling your mind with irrelevant information.

REFLECTION

This chapter focused on powering your mind and perhaps increased your awareness of wasted time while dwelling on trivial tasks.

1. **How often do you take time to clear your mind?**

2. **What techniques will you adopt to increase the regularity at which you clear your mind?**

3. **What actions can you take to reduce the time spent on your phone?**

6. POWER YOUR BREATHING

Twenty Thousand. That's how many breaths an average adult takes every day. It is a subconscious habit and a fundamental of life. In, out, in, out, in, out.

On the face of it, breathing seems a relatively straightforward process, when in fact, that couldn't be further from reality. Your respiratory system provides oxygen to trillions of cells, a complex operation involving every major part of the body. It is a process that fuels you, and this source of energy is often taken for granted, despite its importance.

By focusing on your breathing, you can improve your efficiency and effectiveness when completing regular daily tasks. You can use breathing to clear and focus your mind, with each of the techniques shared in the previous chapter; *Mindfulness, Meditation, and the Mind Dump,* having it at their core.

And how you breathe has varied benefits to your health and wellbeing.

Nasal Breathing

You may have heard or been taught *'in through the nose, out through the mouth'* at a young age. But did you know that by breathing wholly through the nose, you can realise significant health benefits? Firstly, it can reduce the number of contaminants in your body, with your nasal hair acting as a natural air filter. Germs, irritants, and bacteria from the air get trapped on the way in and then expended as you breathe out.

Secondly, there is a natural resistance to airflow as it travels through the narrow nasal cavities. So, as you breathe out through the nose, the oxygen remains in your lungs that little bit longer, increasing the amount that enters the bloodstream. This air also transports naturally produced nitric oxide, a free radical that widens arteries, improves blood flow, and lowers blood pressure.

And finally, the design of your nasal passages warms and humidifies the air as it travels to the lungs, helping avoid cold air on your chest during lower temperatures.

BREATHING TECHNIQUES

Practising breathing exercises at the start of the day is a great way to ground yourself and focus your mind. By taking the time to sit and practise the following techniques, you can teach yourself different ways to breathe for various tasks.

Pursed Lip Breathing

This technique forces you to slow your breathing pace as you concentrate on pursing your lips when exhaling. Particularly beneficial when bending down, heavy lifting, or climbing the stairs, you breathe through the nose for a count of two, then purse your lips and slowly exhale for a count of four.

Belly Breathing (or Diaphragmatic Breathing)

If you are a newcomer to this technique, try lying on your back in the first instance, which helps develop this breathing style properly before you adopt it in a more realistic situation.

Start by lying on your back, your head on a pillow, and a second pillow under your knees to provide further support. Place one hand on your rib cage, with the other resting on your upper chest. You should be able to feel the movement in the diaphragm as you breathe.

Slowly inhale through the nose, allowing your stomach to push your hand out. Exhale, through pursed lips, using your hand to push down on your abdominal muscles, expelling all the air from your lungs. You can make the exercise a little more challenging by placing a book on your stomach.

This technique can bring a feeling of relaxation as you complete your everyday activities.

Equal Breathing

By making your breathing smooth and steady, you can improve balance in both mind and body. In this technique, you inhale and exhale for the same length of time. The difficulty comes in finding a breath length that is not too easy but equally not too challenging. Start with a count of three and progress from there until you find a comfortable timing.

Taking a seated position, inhale and exhale through the nose, counting each breath. Ensure the breaths are even in length, perhaps using a word, or short phrase, to control the pace. To give a more natural feel, add a slight pause between the inhale and exhale. Once you are comfortable practising for around five minutes, you can introduce it to your daily routines. This technique can be particularly beneficial with exercise or Yoga.

Variable Count Breathing

With this technique, each constituent part of the breathing cycle has a different length. A common practice is 3-4-5, where you inhale through the nose for a count of three, hold the breath for four, and then exhale (again through the nose) for a count of five. As you practise regularly, you can increase each stage's count, always ensuring the exhale is longer than the hold, and the inhale is the shortest phase. This technique is a great way to centre yourself at the start of the day.

Lion's Breath

If you take yourself too seriously, then this might not be the technique for you. Considered more unconventional, it may feel very uncomfortable initially, but practising it embraces the positive impact breathing can bring to your health.

Start in a seated position, either on the heels or with your legs crossed. Spread your fingers wide, place your palms on your knees, and inhale deeply through your nose while opening your eyes wide. As you do this, open your mouth wide, stick your tongue out, and bring the tip towards your chin. Exhale through the mouth and contract the front of your throat by making a long '*ha*' sound.

HEALTH AND FITNESS

Your breathing technique is crucial when completing specific tasks, such as lifting, climbing stairs, or exercising. In the case of the latter, it allows you to focus on particular muscle groups and hold the correct form, particularly during resistance workouts, Yoga, or Tai Chi. Let's take a look at the last two exercises and how vital the breathing techniques are.

YOGA

Yoga can be one of the best exercise methods to support your lungs and body health. The constituent parts aim to improve strength and flexibility through a series of movements (poses) coupled with measured and consistent breathing. As you breathe during the poses, the inhale brings a natural tension, which you should embrace before exhaling to get relaxation. Following this pattern will promote a longer exhale when you are looking to relax, be calm and reduce stress.

Many people living with asthma have reported an improvement in symptoms after practising Yoga. By improving your posture, strengthening the chest muscles, and increasing lung capacity, Yoga encourages better breathing.

Building your lung capacity will also help improve fitness during cardio workouts, enabling you to exercise harder for longer. Here are three Yoga poses of varying difficulty that focus on developing strength and breathing.

The Triangle Pose

By opening the chest cavity, this pose allows easy passage of air to the lungs. As you twist the body, it helps massage internal organs, enhancing their ability to remove toxins from the body. One note of caution, if you suffer from back problems, this pose may cause discomfort. Make consideration to this before practising.

1. Start in a standing position, with your legs three feet apart.
2. Turn the right toes outward towards the right wall, and turn your left toes slightly inward.
3. Inhale, pushing your left hip out, and slide both arms to the right, keeping them parallel to the floor.
4. Exhale while rotating only your arms. The left arm is raised upward, with the right hand against your right leg (palm facing outward).

5. Keep your legs strong, and stretch the hands away from each other, bringing the arms into one straight line.
6. Hold the pose for five breaths before returning to the starting position and repeating to the left.

Fish Pose

This pose encourages deep breathing, which provides relief from respiratory disorders, and releases tension from your neck and shoulders. Deep respiration, caused by stretching the lungs, can help distribute oxygen, enhancing your blood circulation.

1. Start by lying on your back with your legs extended and your arms resting alongside your body.
2. Slide your hands (palm down) under your torso, just below the bottom.
3. Press your arms and elbows into the floor, lift your chest, arch your back, and roll onto the crown of the head. It is essential not to use the head or neck to support this posture.
4. Hold the pose for five breaths before releasing back into the starting position.

Seated Twist

By opening the chest, this pose relieves stress and tension held in your back. It increases the supply of oxygen and induces abdominal breathing, enhancing the lungs' capacity.

1. Start in a seated position with your spine erect and your legs stretched out in front.
2. Bend your right knee, and place your right foot outside your left thigh.

3. By bending your left knee, bring your left foot towards your right hip. It is essential not to make this uncomfortable.
4. Slowly raise your left arm, and gently twist your torso to the right, reaching behind with the right arm. If comfortable, place the fingertips of your right hand on the floor.
5. Take five breaths, slowly extended the twist with each one before releasing back to the starting position.

TAI CHI

This chapter's final technique is Tai Chi, a martial arts discipline that focuses on slow, steady movements. The deep, mindful breathing that accompanies the motion is said to achieve balance and harmony and be just what you need to run faster, lift heavier, and go longer.

Tai Chi impacts the entire body through effortless action, providing a steady but impactful workout. The breathing technique used is belly breathing, which focuses on using total lung capacity. Your diaphragm fully inflates the lungs using comparatively slower but deeper breathing, delivering increased oxygen volumes to the bloodstream, and building energy and endurance.

If you are new to Tai Chi, here are three basic movements for you to try.

Broadening The Chest

1. Stand upright with your feet shoulder-width apart, your arms at your side, and weight distributed evenly across both legs.

2. Inhale and raise your arms to a height that feels comfortable but no higher than the shoulders. Keep both your elbows and wrists relaxed.
3. Exhale, allow your shoulders to relax, and with your palms facing each other open your arms, broadening the chest.
4. Inhale and bring your arms back to the middle, continuing to keep the shoulders relaxed.
5. Exhale and bring your arms down to the starting position.

Dancing With Rainbows

1. Stand upright with your feet shoulder-width apart, your arms at your side, and weight distributed evenly across both legs.
2. Inhale, and lift your right arm overhead with the elbow bent. While shifting your weight to the right, extend your left arm out straight, and exhale.
3. Inhale, and in a continuous movement, raise both hands overhead, moving your weight back to the centre.
4. Exhale, and move your weight to the left, mirroring the form previously held on the right.
5. Inhale, and in a continuous movement, raise both hands overhead, moving your weight back to the centre.
6. Exhale and bring your arms down to the starting position.

Circling Arms

1. Stand upright with your feet shoulder-width apart and weight distributed evenly across both legs.

2. Your arms should remain relaxed in front of your body, with your hands crossed and palms facing the torso.
3. Inhale and raise your arms along your body as high as you feel is comfortable, but aiming to reach them overhead.
4. Exhale and lower the arms in a wide, circling motion back to the starting position.

Your body and mind can improve through better breathing, whether through a taught practise or by applying these techniques. Your metabolism can be boosted, along with improved cardiovascular fitness and increased strength and stability. And it's not another task you need to fit into your busy schedule. You breathe every day.

REFLECTION

The last two chapters have shared how breathing can improve physical and mental aptitude.

1. **How often do you focus on your breathing?**
2. **What breathing techniques are you going to try?**
3. **How can you use breathing to help power your mind and body?**

7. POWER YOUR SLEEP

Adults should be taking between seven and nine hours of sleep every night. That is roughly a third of your day spent getting some shut-eye. So, did you get the recommended amount of sleep last night?

If not, you are not alone.

With sleep deprivation more common than you think, around 30% of UK adults have insomnia, with a further 23% managing no more than five hours of sleep a night. That equates to 28 million adults in the UK getting significantly less than the recommended volume of sleep.

When anxiety and stress increase, inconsistent sleeping patterns become the norm. For example, during the Covid-19 pandemic, the number of UK adults reporting insomnia surged. With home and work lives disrupted by lockdown restrictions, homeschooling, and risk of unemployment, anxiety-related problems such as social isolation and child poverty increased. It's not a healthy place to be, as sleep is essential to your existence, helping to maintain your physical and mental fitness.

Tiredness leads to poor food choices, as consumption of unhealthy, sugar-filled snacks and late-night binge eating increases. Over time, these contribute to unhealthy weight gains. Broken sleep patterns raise your blood pressure, a condition that contributes to cardiovascular disease, diabetes, and stroke. An increase in blood pressure may also compromise your immune system, leaving your body unable to rest and repair sufficiently to fight off infections.

The reduced energy levels that tiredness brings leave you at risk of feeling low. In turn, negative thoughts about your lack of sleep play over in your mind. Before you know it, a vicious circle of worry and insomnia ensues. Anxiety becomes a real risk, which can lead to depression.

But don't worry. Through subtle changes, you can introduce habits that make you sleep like a baby.

HOW SLEEP WORKS

Your sleep pattern is controlled by two internal biological mechanisms, the circadian rhythm and homeostasis. Working together, they regulate when you are awake and when you feel sleepy, helping your body operate as efficiently and effectively as possible.

Circadian Rhythm

Your circadian rhythms operate on 24-hour cycles, using your brain's master clock to control many functions within the body. Your sleep-wake cycle is probably the most well-known of these.

Exposure to light during the day results in your body receiving messages that generate alertness, keeping you awake and active. Then, in the evening, your master clock triggers the production of melatonin, the hormone that helps you sleep, and starts sending signals that help you stay asleep during the night. In a perfect environment, this creates restorative rest that allows increased activity while you are awake.

Homeostasis

The great balancing act that your body goes through every hour of every day. Homeostasis is the ability to keep a stable internal environment, regardless of external conditions. After a particular time, your body starts receiving signals that it needs sleep. Known as the sleep drive, the intensity of this feeling gets stronger every hour you are awake, and after a period of deprivation, it will allow more prolonged and deeper sleep.

If you experience any disruption to either of these, your sleep-wake cycle becomes irregular. Natural examples of this are jet lag, as your body adjusts to a new time zone, or night shift working, where sleep occurs when natural light is at its strongest.

You can make some simple changes to improve your sleep.

QUICK WINS

Start by eating a healthier, more nutritional, balanced diet and take regular exercise.

Reducing your mobile phone and television time, particularly close to bedtime, removing the blue light stimuli that make the brain think it is daytime.

Use the techniques from chapter five (Power Your Mind) to clear any thoughts or worries from the day. Perhaps take a warm bath just before bed. By naturally relaxing your mind, you will drift off into a beautiful slumber.

A lack of sleep can lead to irritability, concentration lapses, and tiredness. It becomes too easy to reach for a stimulant, such as caffeine or sugar. Try and avoid excessive consumption of coffee, sugary snacks, or energy drinks, as they can influence both the quantity and quality of sleep.

IT'S ALL ABOUT QUANTITY AND QUALITY

If you are getting your regulation seven to nine hours every night, then that's amazing. Perhaps you are getting the right volume, but what about the quality?

Simply clocking up the hours isn't enough. You need to concentrate as much, if not more, on the quality of your sleep. You want to be leaping out of bed, full of beans, ready to take on the challenges of the day.

Combining a consistent sleeping pattern, where you go to bed and get up as close to the same times each day, with regular exercise and healthy eating, will give you the quantity and quality you need. Your body will thank you for it, and your overall health will reap the benefits.

Improved Concentration

The simple principle is that better sleep provides you with more energy, improving your attention and concentration. A lack of sleep impacts how your body and brain function the following day, perhaps your mind wandering from the task at hand. You will not perform effectively or efficiently when making decisions, assessing risk, or solving problems. Your attention, concentration, and reaction times will be affected, all critical if you drive or operate heavy machinery regularly.

Improved Memory

Falling into a deep sleep allows your brain to process all the information you have received during the day. Your short-term memories are organised and converted into long-term knowledge, which helps you learn and develop problem-solving skills. A great example of this is when you struggle with a problem, and after sleeping on it, quickly find a solution the following day.

Improved Eating Patterns

Logic dictates that if you are awake for longer, your body requires more energy to go about daily life. To provide this energy, you need to consume more, but with tiredness comes poor food choices. You may find difficulty in controlling your appetite, particularly late at night. The kitchen raided under cover of darkness as you search out sugary snacks.

Sleep deprivation also disrupts the hormones that signal hunger (ghrelin) and fullness (leptin), resulting in you making unhealthy food choices. So, making sure you get enough good quality sleep improves your chances of maintaining a healthy weight.

Reduced Risk Of Cardiovascular Disease

In the UK, cardiovascular disease causes more than a quarter of all adult deaths, with a person dying, on average, every three minutes. Getting the correct quality and quantity of sleep is hugely important in reducing your risk of developing heart and circulatory problems, such as high blood pressure, diabetes, and coronary heart disease.

If your sleep pattern becomes disrupted, the body can react as if it is time to wake. The sympathetic nervous system (also responsible for your fight or flight response) stimulates your blood pressure, as it would under normal circumstances. This trigger leads to irregular increases in blood pressure, resulting in higher than average underlying rates, increasing the risks of coronary heart disease and strokes.

Broken sleep can also disrupt insulin regulation and resistance, spiking blood sugar levels, and putting you at risk of developing diabetes.

Improved Immunity

Quality sleep can strengthen your immunity, improving your chances of fighting off illness and disease. As you sleep, your body is resting and repairing the immune system's proteins and cells, which detect and destroy the germs that invade your body. Combined with a healthy diet and regular exercise, sleep creates a more robust body. You can then generate the responses to effectively combat annual viruses, such as the common cold or influenza.

Improved Mental Health

Tiredness can bring with it an increased risk of developing anxiety, depression, or loneliness. You over analysis problems or situations, resulting in things playing on your mind. Under stress, your body releases cortisol, resulting in your energy levels increasing. You struggle to drift off, becoming more stressed by the lack of sleep, which further exacerbates the problem. Getting a good night's sleep relaxes the systems responsible for the stress reactions, positively impacting your mental health in the process.

Improved Mood

When you are tired, you may snap at a loved one or colleague. In some instances, this could be over the most trivial of matters. Better sleep puts you in a positive mood, those around you feel good, and your relationships flourish. Your language is positive, and you develop better reasoning and improved communications skills, all key for strong personal connections.

REFLECTION

Given the numerous benefits of getting the correct quantity and quality of sleep, let's focus on your sleep pattern.

1. How much sleep do you average each night?

2. What actions are you going to take to increase the quality of your sleep?

3. What support do you need to achieve your new sleep pattern?

8. POWER YOUR DETOX

When being healthy, it is vital to take a holistic view of how you are fuelling your body. The natural reaction is to consider what you are consuming, but there is more to it than that, as you will have discovered in the previous chapters.

With toxins being amongst the most significant barriers to improving health, both the amount you are introducing and your body's efficiency in removing them are important considerations. In this chapter, you learn about natural detoxification and explore the effects of three mainstream toxins on the body.

INTERMITTENT FASTING

You may have used over-the-counter detox solutions, which can generate excellent short-term results. But as they tend to focus on calorie restriction, the health benefits are not sustainable, particularly when you return to a regular eating cycle.

A natural way to detox is through intermittent fasting, and while there has been growing popularity in recent years, this alternate eating and fasting cycle is hardly innovative. Over thousands of years, people have been fasting, whether due to scarcity or following religious beliefs. At varying times during the year, Islam (Ramadan), Christianity (Lent), and Judaism (Yom Kippur) all mandate periods of not eating.

You naturally fast when feeling unwell, as often you lose your appetite when fighting viral or bacterial infections.

While during sleep, cells repair and regenerate, removing waste from the body—a natural fasting cycle only broken by your first meal of the day. Over time, breakfast, or the food that BREAKS the FAST, has become a traditional morning meal, but this doesn't have to be the case. Breaking a fast can happen later in the day, as you will discover.

All of this points to the fact that your body is well equipped to handle extended periods of not eating, despite years of evolutionary change and food availability being better than ever.

You can naturally extend the time you don't eat, perhaps not taking your first meal until later in the day or not consuming food after a specific time. This can be challenging at first, as you will instinctively feel hungry at your regular mealtimes, and cutting out the late-night hot drinks can be difficult. But over time, your body becomes accustomed to the changes. You could consider slowly extending your fasting window over a few weeks to make the transition easier.

How Intermittent Fasting Works

As you travel through your fasting window, your blood glucose level drops, slowing or even stopping insulin production. Your body reacts by burning stored carbohydrates, and once that stock has depleted, it moves onto your fat reserves. So, the longer you go without introducing food or calorific drinks into the body, the better the health benefits. The introduction of even the smallest amount of food (or calorific beverages, such as tea, coffee, or soft drinks) triggers your metabolism, effectively resetting the clock and preventing the full benefit from being achieved.

The Benefits Of Intermittent Fasting

People cite having more energy during the fast and feel both physically and mentally healthier. As you increase the fasting window, you are likely to eat fewer meals, possibly reducing your calorie intake in the process. Some choose to eat the same number of meals in less time or increase portion sizes. Either way, your body will burn more fat as you are without food for an extended period.

Because of this, weight loss is often the most high-profile benefit to intermittent fasting. An increased metabolic rate burns more abdominal fat, reducing the risk of developing several diseases. Breaking down fat enhances hormone functionality, lowers insulin levels, and increases noradrenaline, which results in increased energy levels. You also find it easier to maintain muscle mass, which is a challenge if you follow a calorie-restrictive eating pattern.

When you go without food, your body will start a cellular repair process known as *Autophagy.* This self-preservation mechanism recycles and removes damaged and dysfunctional cells, cleaning debris from your body and improving its functional effectiveness. Cells and tissue get damaged through oxidative stress when your body has an imbalance between free radicals and antioxidants. By fasting, you allow your body to neutralise the effects, reducing the risk of developing several diseases, including cancer and Alzheimer's Disease, and slowing the signs of ageing. For this reason, fasting has now become very popular in anti-ageing circles

Intermittent fasting can also help you reduce inflammation and regulate blood sugar levels, with the latter reducing the risk of developing Type 2 diabetes. Both these effects also help lower the risk of developing high blood pressure, cholesterol, and triglycerides, all chronic conditions linked with cardiovascular disease.

Your mental health will also improve, as neurological health benefits from the combination of reduced oxidative stress and inflammation, coupled with the increase in insulin resistance. Fasting also increases a hormone called a brain-derived neurotrophic factor, which reduces the risk of developing depression and other neurological problems. With management the only current option, short-term fasts may alleviate some symptoms of Alzheimer's Disease.

As you can see, intermittent fasting can create harmony in your body and mind, and through straightforward changes, puts a new healthier lifestyle within your grasp.

Intermittent Fasting Options

There are several straightforward intermittent fasting regimes that you can try. All involve abstaining from food for a set period before eating regularly and, most importantly, healthily. If you are considering following a fasting regime, remember that certain methods may suit you better. Take time to find the right one, considering how you can fit it into your lifestyle, when you can commit to eating regularly, and who else in the household may be affected. In the long term, fasting can be easier to follow than calorie-restrictive diets, so make sure you try different techniques before dismissing it entirely.

Hourly Fasting Windows

The rules for this style of fasting are simple. Decide on, and adhere to, the same fasting window every day. You could start with a ten-hour fast, let's say 8:00 p.m. to 6:00 a.m., and build from there. By increasing the fasting window by an hour every week, you can combat the hunger pains while continually improving the health benefits. Within a few months, you can reach the 16:8 method, where you fast for 16 hours and feed for eight.

By starting with a smaller fasting window, you can build it into your regular sleeping pattern, working back from breakfast time to determine when the last meal is in the evening. Only once the window exceeds 12 hours will you require more flexibility regarding when and how you fast. A common approach is to skip breakfast and start eating later in the day, perhaps finishing around 7:00 p.m.

Fasting for longer than 14 hours can increase the risk of women developing hormone imbalance, which can affect the menstrual cycle, fertility, and bone health. Seeking professional medical advice is always advisable for any gender before starting a fast.

Daily Fasting Windows

Another popular and well-known approach to fasting is the 5:2 diet, where you consume healthy meals for five days and restrict calories on the remaining two. With restricted days seeing as little as 500 calories consumed, you should always seek to have one healthy day between your fasting days. You may find it easier to adopt this method by keeping a regular weekly cycle, perhaps fasting on Tuesday and Friday.

A more radical approach is choosing to fast every other day, where you eat what you want on feeding days while avoiding solid foods altogether on fast days. While you may consume the same or more calories than the 5:2 approach, fasting for three or four days a week may not be suitable for everyone.

Extreme Fasting Windows

The Eat-Stop-Eat Fast involves you consuming no food for 24 hours, maybe fasting from breakfast to breakfast, perhaps even twice a week. During fasting periods, non-calorific drinks, such as water or hot drinks without milk, are allowed and, on feeding days, you should follow a regular pattern of healthy eating. With side effects such as fatigue, irritability, and headaches, this approach can be very challenging and, for this reason, is probably not for a beginner.

You could also try The Warrior Diet, or 20 hours fast, which allows you to eat minimal amounts during the fasting window. Often small servings of raw fruit and vegetables are followed by one large meal at night, which followers of this method believe is better suited to your circadian rhythm (or sleep pattern). By having only one large meal, you need to ensure you are getting a balanced diet, so include plenty of vegetables, proteins, and healthy fats, along with carbohydrates. Possible downsides to this method are missing recommended fibre levels and feeling uncomfortable after eating a large meal in the evening.

Meal Skipping

By choosing to skip a meal each day, it is a very flexible approach to fasting. It feels more natural as you react to both hunger levels and time constraints, making it suitable for beginners. When you do feel hungry, always eat a balanced healthy meal, and avoid those sugary snacks.

Earlier in the chapter, you learnt that a significant benefit to fasting is the recycling and regeneration of cells by removing waste and toxins, resulting in your body functioning more effectively. Unless you live a 100% clean life, which most people don't, you will be introducing varying levels of toxins into your body. As with anything unhealthy, the more you put in, the longer it takes to remove, which can lead to a build-up of toxins, ultimately harming your overall health.

As you will see in the next chapter, staying hydrated has many benefits, including the efficient removal of toxins from your body. Alcohol, caffeine, and energy drinks are three commonly consumed products that can reduce hydration levels, impacting your health and vitality.

Remember, you don't have to be 100% clean living every day. Everything in moderation is acceptable, but understanding the effect these products can have on your health means you can make informed decisions and ensure more good days than bad.

ALCOHOL

You wake up after a big night out, your mouth dry and head throbbing. Classic signs of dehydration, or as it is more commonly known, a hangover. What you may not be aware of is that this all starts from the first sip of your pint, glass of wine, or gin and tonic.

The occasional alcoholic drink isn't a cause for concern, but when it becomes more regular or in excess, the cumulative effect on your body eventually takes its toll. With the current guidance on alcohol consumption in the UK being no more than 14 units a week, you may consider spreading your drinking over three or more days and always include alcohol-free days. If you are looking to reduce your alcohol consumption, try using the *Beat The Week* technique described in chapter 4 (Power Your Habits) to increase your drink-free days.

Although adhering to the guidelines may have minimal impact on your overall health, you are still introducing toxins to your body that need removing as effectively and efficiently as possible. Increasing your intake at times of stress or excessive consumption in one session (binge-drinking) can result in a build-up over time, leading to some severe conditions and illness.

Pancreatitis

Excessive alcohol consumption can lead to inflammation of the pancreas. The abnormal activation of digestive enzymes causes swelling, resulting in severe complications if it develops into a long-term condition.

Liver

The liver is one of the organs that help to break down and remove toxins from your body. Excessive and consistent alcohol consumption can disrupt the process, increasing the risk of chronic liver inflammation and liver disease. The inflammation causes scarring, known as cirrhosis, which can damage the liver, resulting in inefficient removal of toxins. If left untreated, the inflammation can lead to life-threatening liver disease.

Blood Sugar

Damage or inflammation of both the pancreas and liver puts you at risk of hypoglycaemia (low blood sugar). With your pancreas regulating insulin use and your body's response to glucose, damage can also put you at risk of hyperglycaemia (too much sugar in the blood). Unable to manage and balance your blood sugar results in complications and side effects relating to diabetes. If you suffer from either hypoglycaemia or diabetes, you should always avoid excessive amounts of alcohol.

Central Nervous System

You will see the impact on the central nervous system through how you speak, move and think. Slurred speech is one of the first signs you have had one too many, with the alcohol affecting communications between your body and brain. Coordination becomes more challenging, with you perhaps losing your balance more quickly, and your brain struggles to form long-term memories. Your ability to think is impaired, and decision-making becomes less rational and more impulsive.

Continual excessive alcohol consumption can lead to longer-term conditions, such as frontal lobe damage, which adversely affects emotional response, judgement, and the ability to form short-term memory.

Digestive System

Perhaps not immediately apparent how they are connected, but alcohol consumption can harm your digestive system. Worryingly the side effects only become evident once damage to the tissue in your digestive tract has occurred. Your intestines become unable to digest food and absorb nutrients effectively, with malnutrition occurring in extreme cases. Drinking alcohol frequently can also increase the risk of developing cancer of the mouth, throat, oesophagus, colon, or liver.

Cardiovascular System

Chronic alcohol consumption can affect your heart and lungs, increasing the risk of developing cardiovascular problems and diseases. Common conditions include high blood pressure, irregular heartbeat, stroke, heart attack, and heart disease. Anaemia can also develop as alcohol impacts your ability to absorb vitamins and minerals from food effectively.

Reproductive Health

A common misconception is that alcohol lowers your inhibitions, making the bedroom more fun! The reality is quite different, with erectile dysfunction, low libido, and reduced testosterone regularly suffered by men. For women, the menstrual cycle can be affected, increasing the risk of infertility. The risk of premature birth, miscarriage, or stillbirth increases with excessive drinking during pregnancy, as does the risk of an unborn child developing learning difficulties, poor emotional wellbeing, or long-term health problems.

Skeletal And Muscle Systems

Long-term alcohol use can reduce bone density and strength, increase fracture risk, and slow the healing process. Later in life, this can lead to osteoporosis or arthritis, both of which can restrict movement and make it challenging to maintain a healthy weight. In turn, this can contribute to the risk of developing Type 2 diabetes and cardiovascular disease.

Muscles can also become weaker, with cramps (due to dehydration) becoming a regular occurrence. In extreme cases, atrophy, more commonly known as muscle wasting, can occur.

Immune System

Heavy drinking reduces your body's natural immune system, with your immune cells and fine hairs in your lungs become damaged through excessive alcohol consumption. Once these are damaged, your body finds it challenging to clear pathogens from your airway, making it more difficult to fight off germs and viruses.

Addiction

Developing a physical and emotional dependency on alcohol can often be triggered by stressful situations in your personal or professional life. Common symptoms include anxiety, nervousness, nausea, and tremors, with more severe problems being high blood pressure, an irregular heartbeat, and heavy perspiration. It is essential to seek professional help to break any addiction, as withdrawal can be difficult and life-threatening.

CAFFEINE

Millions of people reach for caffeine first thing in the morning, and with over 2,000 shops, the UK consumes around 95 million cups of coffee every day. Caffeine is perceived as a quick fix for low energy levels, not only at the start but at various points during the day.

You may not be a coffee person and might be sitting there thinking about skipping the rest of the section. Unfortunately, there is bad news, as caffeine is present in many foods and drinks, including chocolate, energy drinks, and some cereals. And that British standard, a cup of tea. Yes, that's got it too. Even when you reach for the medicine cabinet, some headache tablets will be covertly topping up your caffeine levels.

Caffeine has no nutritional value and can be mildly addictive, so think twice before having that third or fourth cup of coffee. Your body can also build a tolerance, forcing you to increase consumption to get the same energy boost as before, accelerating the adverse impact on your body in the process. If you are trying to reduce your intake, then approach it slowly to minimise the risk of withdrawal symptoms. These are often as bad as some of the following issues caused by excessive levels.

Central Nervous System

When caffeine reaches your brain, you start to feel more alert. For this reason, it makes an effective ingredient in medicines that treat drowsiness, headaches, and migraines. Despite this, excessive caffeine can be the root cause of suffering headaches in the first place.

Cardiovascular And Digestion

Caffeine is absorbed via your stomach and can take up to two hours to reach peak levels in your bloodstream. During this time, you are raising your blood pressure for a short while, increasing adrenaline, and putting a temporary block on hormones that naturally widen arteries. For those with heart murmurs or hypertension (high blood pressure), caffeine can put added pressure on your body, as it forces your heart to pump harder.

Other digestive issues, including heartburn, acid reflux, or ulcers, can be caused by increased stomach acid levels due to excessive caffeine consumption. You may find reducing caffeine, even if you have no plans to remove it altogether, will help.

Liver

Your body doesn't store caffeine, which is why you may reach for another coffee mid-afternoon to give you that quick energy hit. Before caffeine enters the bloodstream, it is metabolised by the liver, with any excess leaving the body almost immediately, as urine. This process temporarily impairs blood sugar levels, which in turn affects other bodily functions. With the body then depleting liver glycogen to compensate, your energy levels reduce, and you are back to square one.

Bone Density And Strength

A large amount of caffeine can contribute to osteoporosis, a condition that weakens your bones. Caffeine interferes with calcium absorption and metabolism, which slows your bones' development and healing, making a speedy recovery from breaks and fractures challenging.

The muscles around your bones can also be affected, with twitches occurring if you have consumed excessive amounts of caffeine, and withdrawal can result in muscle ache.

Reproduction

If you are trying to or have successfully got pregnant, you may consider reducing caffeine consumption. Excessive amounts of caffeine can interfere with oestrogen (the pregnancy hormone) and your metabolism. While pregnant, your baby's heart rate and metabolism can be stimulated by caffeine in the bloodstream that crosses the placenta. With above-average levels of caffeine, this can, in some instances, increase the risk of miscarriage and slow foetal growth.

Overdose

In extreme cases, people have overdosed on caffeine, resulting in hallucinations, vomiting, and becoming easily confused. One of the most common reasons is excessive consumption of energy drinks, and there is more about these later in the chapter.

Withdrawal

Your body, and particularly your brain, can build a tolerance to the effect of caffeine, as it does with any stimulant. If you are consuming excessive levels, then you should handle reducing or withdrawing caffeine with care. Going cold turkey can cause headaches as your brain struggles to compensate for the reduction in caffeine, with anxiety, irritability, and drowsiness, being other common symptoms.

Recommended Daily Levels

The equivalent of four small cups from your favourite coffee house is considered safe, but who has small serves? Those large cups mean you've possibly reached your limit after the second trip of the day. And it's not just the cup size you need to consider. Different beverages, with varying grounds of coffee, can dramatically change the amount of caffeine. Even a simple espresso can vary in intensity, resulting in inconsistent caffeine levels.

Decaffeinated Products

With a much more comprehensive range available, including many teas and coffees, moving to decaffeinated drinks is a straightforward way to reduce your caffeine intake. Be mindful though, as a common misconception is that decaffeinated means that it is entirely free from caffeine, and unfortunately, this isn't always the case. Let's take decaffeinated coffee as an example, which, even after processing, has around 3% of the caffeine remaining in the beans. That's up to seven milligrams in your decaffeinated latte to go.

While this section has focused on the impact of excessive consumption, coffee in moderation is an excellent antioxidant source. And even moving to decaffeinated products will not significantly impact the benefits. A decaffeinated coffee can contain anywhere between 85-100% of its full-strength cousin's antioxidant levels.

ENERGY DRINKS

Their advertising is everywhere. It's a multi-billion pound industry, and if popularity is a sign of effectiveness, energy drinks appear to be doing their job. But energy drinks have serious caffeine content, with some single serves containing as much as two or three cups of coffee. And you already know about the potential negative effect that could have on your body.

Ingredients also include additives like guarana and ginseng, and while added to amplify the energy boost, they can also magnify the adverse effects of caffeine. These energy drinks often contain large amounts of sugar, in some instances over ten teaspoons. Increasing the risk of developing high blood pressure and high cholesterol, both linked to obesity and cardiovascular disease.

Despite legislation back in 2010 banning alcoholic energy drinks, it remains a common trend for late-night venues to offer mixed drinks. By combining a stimulant with an antidepressant in this way, you stay awake for longer and perhaps consume more alcohol, increasing the adverse effects on your body.

A quick fix for fatigue, but linked to obesity, high blood pressure, and cardiovascular disease. Just one energy drink can provide more than the recommended daily allowance for both sugar and caffeine. There are plenty of healthy alternatives that you could consider.

HEALTHY ALTERNATIVES

Drink Water
Stay hydrated by drinking a glass of water when you wake up, with meals, and before, during, and after workouts. Refer to chapter nine to find out more about the additional benefits of staying hydrated.

Balanced Healthy Eating
If your meals include all the principal fuels for your body, particularly protein and carbohydrates, there is little need to

boost energy in other ways. Check out chapter 10 to add power to your plate.

Vitamin Supplements

Consider increasing energy levels through high-quality supplements or add more vitamin and mineral-rich foods, such as fresh fruits, vegetables, nuts, and yogurt, to your diet.

Move Regularly

When you feel tired, move your body. It is one of the best ways to boost energy levels, despite it being a little counter-intuitive. Exercise increases serotonin and endorphin levels, and these happy hormones help you feel better, revitalised, and energised. Baseline energy levels will improve the more regularly you exercise.

REFLECTION

1. **How many units of alcohol or caffeinated drinks do you consume in a typical week?**

2. **What other foodstuffs are you consuming that may contain caffeine?**

3. **What action can you take to reduce or remove toxins, such as caffeine or alcohol, from your diet?**

9. POWER YOUR HYDRATION

Your body requires a steady supply of water throughout the day. Bodily functions, such as breathing, sweating, and urinating, deplete your reserves constantly. You can even lose up to a litre of fluid while you sleep.

60% of your body is made up of water, so staying hydrated is incredibly important for your overall health. Your brain and heart are 73% water, with your lungs even higher, at 83%. Your skin contains 64% water, muscles and kidneys 79%, and your bones are nearly one third water. Every essential organ needs you to replenish your water supply.

Consider starting your day with a glass of water before you grab breakfast. It not only replaces the fluids lost through sleeping but kick-starts your metabolism too.

But just how much should you be drinking?

RECOMMENDED DAILY CONSUMPTION

A well-recognised approach to staying hydrated is the eight by eight method. Drink eight, eight-ounce glasses of water, the equivalent of a two-litre bottle, regularly across the day. To get a reminder, set notifications on your phone. It's a fantastic way of hitting the numbers.

An alternative method is to drink one litre of water for every 20 kilograms you weigh. For an average UK male, this equates to four litres. For an average UK female, three and a half litres. These are both significantly higher than the eight-by-eight method.

You may not realise, but up to 20% of your water consumption can come from the food you consume. As with several other influences affecting hydration, it is crucial to strike the right balance and adjust your volumes accordingly.

INTERNAL AND EXTERNAL INFLUENCES

Diet
A healthy balanced approach to the food and drink you consume will help your hydration. Drinking caffeinated beverages, like coffee, result in you losing more water through urination. Dehydration also increases if you consume high quantities of salty, spicy, or sugary foods. Replacing them with water-rich fruit and vegetables, such as cucumber, strawberries, and watermelon, improves the hydration level in your diet.

Environment
It's probably not a surprise, but you require more regular hydration in hot, humid, or dry areas. Experiencing high temperatures or being outdoors result in increased fluid loss. Living in the mountains or at a high altitude can also result in increased water consumption. The more rapid breathing required in these conditions contributes to more significant fluid loss. In general, during the warmer months, you will sweat more. Constantly adjust your water intake accordingly.

Exercise And Activity
If you are active during the day, whether walking or standing for long periods, you will naturally lose more water. Exercising or intense activity accelerates the depletion rate

further, so take more water on board, before, during, and after training.

Health

Underlying health conditions, such as diabetes, cystic fibrosis, or kidney disease, can cause dehydration. Vomiting or diarrhoea, associated symptoms of infection or fever, result in rapid fluid loss, and medicinal diuretics may cause excessive water loss through urination. You should drink plenty of fluids when you feel unwell.

Another cause of dehydration can be stress, and stress can also be a contributing factor to dehydration. A vicious cycle begins as your body fails to function correctly without hydration, which leads to stress. The anxiety experienced leads to further reductions in fluid intake, worsening the impact of dehydration.

Pregnancy

With the foetus placing additional demands on the body, there is a risk of dehydration as the need for nutrients increases. Further hydration issues can be caused by morning sickness, as the body loses fluids quickly and fails to absorb water efficiently. With the body doing the work for two, or more, drinking extra water ensures hydration levels are satisfactory.

WATER QUALITY

Cold running water straight from the tap is easily accessible and readily available for most people. In the UK, the domestic supply is safe to drink but still contains low levels of contaminants. The residue of copper, or lead in older pipes, can be picked up as the water finds its way to your home. The cleaning process can result in chlorine by-products being present, and there are modern risks to contend with, such as microplastics and contamination from pharmaceutical products.

Now more readily available and easier to use, domestic water filters have risen in popularity in recent years. You can choose one to suit your needs, with independently tested, credible brands providing a choice of solutions for any budget. You can install under-sink options that feed straight from the water supply or have water jugs with recyclable filters. The choice is yours. But choose wisely.

Take account of the ease of installation and required maintenance, as poor practices can impact water quality dramatically. The risks include removing all minerals and possible bacterial growth due to poor maintenance. Both can be as detrimental to your health as any of the contamination risks from the domestic supply.

BENEFITS OF HYDRATION

Fluid loss of 2% equates to around two kilos of body weight for an average UK adult. Your regular daily routine may account for this reduction, showing how important hydration is to function effectively during the day.

Maximise Physical Performance

Staying hydrated during intense exercise is particularly important. Losing just 2% of your body's fluids results in a noticeable impact on physical performance. That is just over a litre to an average adult, which is easily lost while sleeping. Losing this relatively small amount alters your body temperature, reduces motivation, and increases fatigue. Exercising becomes more challenging, both physically and mentally. Stay hydrated to perform at your absolute best.

Energy Levels And Brain Function

Mild dehydration, defined as the loss of just one or two litres of water, can impair brain function. Fluid loss at this level can affect your mood, the ability to concentrate and increases the occurrence of headaches or migraine symptoms. It can be detrimental to working memory and increase anxiety and fatigue.

Control Your Appetite

Your body is easily confused, often thinking it needs food when in fact, you are dehydrated. Therefore, the more hydrated you are, the less likely you are to overeat, with hunger pains subdued by drinking water. Your food choices will also impact your appetite, with increased consumption of water-rich foods such as fruits and vegetables preventing snacking between meals.

Healthy Skin

Dehydrated skin is more likely to appear dry and wrinkled. Increasing your fluid intake will help keep a healthier complexion and is often championed by anti-ageing groups. Water is not a miracle beauty product though, with over-hydrated skin still having evidence of fine lines and wrinkles.

Kidney And Bowel Function

Being fully hydrated results in your body operating in a highly effective manner. Your kidneys purify your blood and remove waste products efficiently through urination. A strong-smelling or dark urine highlights the need for hydration, with long-term low-level dehydration leaving you susceptible to increased risk of kidney stones or urinary tract infections.

Drinking plenty of water also supports a healthy digestive system, with dehydration leading to uncomfortable issues such as constipation. Focus on gut health is increasing and can be linked to both physical and mental fitness. To create the perfect environment to keep your gut healthy, you should combine the correct hydration levels with your recommended fibre intake. The average adult in the UK eats 20g of fibre daily, around 70% of the recommended levels. Increasing the amount of beans, fruit, and lentils in your diet improves fibre levels.

To achieve improved hydration, follow these three simple rules. Your body will love you for it.

1. Drink regularly during the day.
2. When you feel hungry, drink water first.
3. Increase water intake when exercising or temperatures are high.

REFLECTION

To close out this chapter, reflect on your current approach to hydration and how you can improve it.

1. On average, how much water do you currently drink daily?

2. What water-rich foods (fruit and vegetables) do you currently consume?

3. How can you increase both your fluid and water-rich food intake?

10. POWER YOUR PLATE

By definition, everyone is on a diet. You habitually eat certain types of food and consume particular drinks to fuel your body. But over time, the word diet has become associated with restrictive eating patterns, with only one goal, to deliver short-term weight loss.

You cannot sustain these programmes in the long term, with weight gains post-diet often more significant than the original loss. It's a case of no carbohydrates, no fat, and no fun. Through constantly watching your weight and what you consume, these restrictive eating patterns can create a cycle of negativity. Your stress levels increase when you don't hit your numbers, slowing your metabolism further. Lacking energy, you will struggle to get fired up for the challenges ahead, and these yo-yo diets can cause more harm than good in the longer term.

Weight-loss or restrictive dieting is limiting, foods are in, or foods are out. There are no ifs, buts, or maybes. You have your goal, a target weight that is the only focus, with no consideration for how you feel, physically, mentally, or emotionally. It is black and white, with no grey, and this lack of flexibility can result in you falling out of love with your diet.

Healthy eating should be intuitive, flexible, and fun. Allowing consideration for how food and drink nurture your mind, body, and soul helps deliver sustainable results. It is about making an informed choice, embracing that grey area as there is no right or wrong. You are in charge of your options, so whether you want to share that fantastic pizza while out with friends or refuse dessert because you are full, make your choice feel good.

MINDFUL EATING

From chapter five, you know that mindfulness anchors you in the present. It can be a technique that you apply to any task or activity, including mealtimes. As you eat your meal, take a moment, and allow the food to arouse your senses. Be mindful, even before you eat, thinking about what foods you are buying or preparing. You will nourish your body effectively and efficiently by making healthier choices.

Here are some straightforward techniques to help you eat more mindfully.

Take Time

Your stomach and brain have a connection and are constantly sending messages to each other. Despite this, your brain doesn't start reacting to food immediately. It may be 20 minutes into your meal before you realise you are feeling full. Slow down and be mindful about every mouthful. Give the brain time to recognise the amount of food you are consuming. Take small bites, and chew thoroughly before diving back in. Even try putting your knife and fork down between mouthfuls. Turn every mealtime into an experience.

Secret Snacking

One of the biggest challenges to healthy eating is *secret snacking*. The risk of poor food choices elevates outside of traditional mealtimes, as you reach for food without recognising the nutritional impact it may or may not have. It might be those office birthday cakes or nibbling on leftovers. It's a minefield you need to avoid.

Try keeping a food diary, writing down everything you consume. When you see it in black and white, you will be surprised how many covert calories you are consuming. Being mindful of this will improve your choices, even removing regular daily snacking from your diet permanently.

Food Or No Food

When you feel hungry, it's easy to grab a convenient snack. Autopilot takes over, and you decide without thinking. You may find a walk or drinking a glass of water will satisfy any urge you have to eat. Even if you arrive at the decision you are famished, consider all your options and use all your senses to arrive at the right choice. It is the difference between devouring an actual orange or a chocolate one. And deep down, you know which is more nutritional.

Table Manners

You move at one hundred miles per hour, racing to complete your tasks for the day. Convenience food is on the rise, and you can easily fall into the trap of eating anywhere but at the dining table. Travelling in the car, your desk at work, even public transport have all become acceptable places to consume food and drink.

By not taking a clean break, your brain fails to recognise mealtimes, increasing the risk of making poor choices. Eating at a table or a different area at work improves your chances of considering what food and drink you consume. You make better decisions and have a more enjoyable food experience.

Focus On The Food (And The Family)

Creating rituals, particularly around mealtimes, is difficult. Working adults, with flexible hours, may very rarely eat together. Throw the kids into the mix, and it becomes even more challenging. Taking time to eat as a family or with partners is an opportunity to appreciate both the food and company. Switch off your phones, computers, and television to facilitate conversations about each other's day. While you concentrate on talking and listening, you are not eating and allowing your brain to decide whether you are full or not.

HEALTHY EATING

You now know everyone is on a diet, restrictive eating is not sustainable, and mindful eating can naturally support healthy eating.

But what is healthy eating? And how can you add power to your plate?

No single food contains all the essential vitamins and nutrients that your body needs to stay healthy. In the UK, there are five main food groups to consider for your diet (indicative proportions in brackets):

Fruit and Vegetables (41%)

Starchy carbohydrates, such as potatoes, bread, rice, and pasta (38%)

Dairy and alternatives (8%)

Proteins, such as beans, pulses, fish, eggs, and meat (12%)

Oils and spreads (1%)

Healthy eating should provide you with energy balance, which in its simplest form means calories in equals calories out. Closely following the five main food groups' suggested proportions provides the balance to complete everyday tasks. Your body functions effectively and efficiently through a healthy balanced diet. Among others, the respiratory and cardiovascular systems rely on healthy energy reserves, and consuming a wide range of foods helps them function.

TASTE THE RAINBOW

Rainbows are one of nature's wonders, a spectrum of colour that stretches into infinity. To step up to the challenge of introducing a healthier balance to your food choices, use the rainbow for inspiration. The positive energy created by the band of colour instantly removes the negativity of the rain that preceded it.

By creating a rainbow on your plate, you can instantly improve the provision of the nutrients and vitamins required to function at full capacity. You can generate energy through minor changes, fixing many aches, pains, or problems in the process. You are using this rainbow to remove negative influences and feelings from your diet.

Adding more colourful fruits and vegetables to your diet introduces a broad spectrum of vitamins and antioxidants. The healthier you are, the better you feel, and these nutrients help protect your body against cancer, heart disease, and other conditions. You improve your overall wellbeing, with even the slightest change enhancing brain health and protection against ageing.

Each colour has its nutritional benefits, and the ratio of vegetables to fruit is important. Fruit contains more natural sugar and calories and should form a lower proportion of your diet than vegetables. In the UK, the recommendation is a ratio of around 60:40 in favour of vegetables. On this basis, using the UK's five portions a day guideline, three should be vegetables.

Introducing a rainbow to your diet will help maintain a healthy weight and facilitate the absorption of a comprehensive range of nutrients. Let's take a look at the benefits of each colour.

Red

Containing antioxidants that reduce the risk of developing plaque in the arteries, hypertension, and high cholesterol, red fruit and vegetables protect our heart. They can reduce the risk of different cancer types, including prostate, and support brain function improvement.

To increase consumption, add radishes, red cabbage, or beetroot to a leafy salad, or improve your intake of berries, such as strawberries, raspberries, or cranberries. For a great snack, try a fruit salad with red grapes, pomegranate, and watermelon.

Orange And Yellow

High in vitamin A, these are packed with nutrients to protect your nervous system, promote eye health and prevent heart disease. Playing an essential role in maintaining skin health, they also boost your immune system and help build bone density and strength.

You can slow roast some carrots, butternut squash, and sweet potatoes before blitzing them with vegetable stock to make a hearty soup. Orange, grapefruit, pineapple, and mango make a great tropical fruit salad and swap your sugary snacks for a yellow apple variety such as Golden Delicious.

Green

The superstars of the rainbow, green fruits and vegetables protect your eye health by lowering the risk of age-related macular degeneration. Green leafy vegetables contain folic acid, hugely crucial for pregnant women, as it reduces the risk of congenital disabilities and hormone imbalance. The essential nutrients in these fruits and vegetables can reduce the risk of cancer and low-density lipoprotein (bad cholesterol), plus regulates digestion and improves the immune system.

Spinach or lettuce can form the base for a salad, and broccoli, cabbage, or courgette make great soups. Avocado is an excellent side for a breakfast or brunch, and a fruit cocktail of green apple, kiwi, lime juice, and green grapes is a refreshing change to yoghurt.

Blue And Purple

Blue or purple fruit and vegetables can help prevent heart disease, stroke, and cancer. They can also help improve memory, promote healthy aging, protect urinary tract health, and regulate digestion.

Perhaps not as widely seen as some of the other colours, you can add aubergine to a vegetable traybake or replace green cabbage with a purple variety. Add some blackberries, blueberries, plums, or raisins to your snack options to increase your intake.

White

Containing nutrients that are known to lower the level of low-density lipoprotein (bad cholesterol), white fruit and vegetables can help regulate high blood pressure and provide an immune-boosting effect on your body. In some instances, they may reduce the risk of colon, prostate, and breast cancer.

Try potato and onion as the base ingredient for soups, and complement your traditional Sunday roast with cauliflower or turnip. Start your day with banana rather than cereal, or grab a pear as an alternative to a chocolate bar.

PLANT-BASED EATING

The popularity of flexitarian, vegetarian and vegan diets is growing exponentially. Millions of adults in the UK are actively increasing the proportion of plant-based eating in their daily routine. Driven by the increased availability and quality, the market is big business, with the UK worth an estimated £700m per annum (2020).

There are some common misconceptions about this type of eating, which we will explore later, but first, do humans suit a plant-based diet?

You will all know the three primary classifications of animals; *herbivore, omnivore, and carnivore*. Based on what they eat, herbivorous animals, like the elephant, cows, and deer, chew on grass or rip leaves from trees. Their carnivorous cousins, the predators such as big cats, sharks, and spiders, seek out other animals as food. Finally, the omnivores, like bears, raccoons, and dogs, choose to search out meat or plants.

So, what label would you give humans?

The typical answer is that humans are omnivores. After all, the majority of people still eat a combination of meat and plants.

Physiologically, this is true. Humans can get all the nutrients needed for a healthy lifestyle from meat and plants, and your body can consume and process both food types.

Behaviourally, humans exhibit omnivorous traits, actively consuming both plant and animal products by choice.

Anatomically, humans have more in common with herbivores than either carnivores or omnivores. You chew your food into smaller chunks of food, with saliva softening it before swallowing. True meat-eaters can devour large pieces immediately, and have razor-sharp canine teeth, unlike humans. The human jaw has multi-lateral movement, allowing food to be ground rather than powerfully bitten down upon—another herbivorous trait.

As you move down the body, the chemical makeup suggests a herbivorous digestive system. Human saliva breaks down plant food's complex carbohydrates into simple sugars. The acid contained in the stomach is at a lower concentration, strong enough to break down plant protein easily, but finds meat products more challenging. Human digestion is naturally slow, with food travelling through an intestine that can measure around fifteen feet in length, the equivalent of two and a half Yoga mats. It is an environment that is better suited to the breakdown of plant-derived foods, with any meat beginning to rot in the gut before digestion is complete.

Another indicator of herbivorous anatomy is the inability to produce Vitamin C naturally, an essential nutrient absorbed from foods or supplements to ensure your body functions correctly. Both carnivores and omnivores produce it naturally, perhaps suggesting evolution has made humans more herbivorous.

More anatomical signals that humans are more herbivorous by nature are hands designed to gather, cooling through sweating, not panting, and sipping, not lapping, water and drinks.

In summary, based on physiological and behavioural traits, humans are omnivores, choosing to follow a mixed diet. But anatomically, humans are herbivores, able to decide to pursue a more plant-based path if preferred.

Despite continual availability, daily servings of fruit and vegetables have reduced by up to two-thirds. Over time animals have become actively farmed rather than hunted. Meat is more readily available, meaning your consumption of antioxidants and nutrients from plant-based food is now a fraction of that seen in previous hunter-gatherer species.

This section is not trying to convince you of a specific path to follow regarding healthy eating but hopefully provides you with, excuse the pun, food for thought.

There are several myths about plant-based eating, many coming from general misunderstanding or misinformation. Quickly circulating inaccurate nutritional information or product development does not help matters. One constant is that diversity in your diet is essential, and here are some myth busters for you to consider.

Plant-Based Is Not Vegan

A plant-based diet means that a higher proportion of your diet comes from fruit, vegetables, and nuts. Increasing the amount does not mean you have to become vegan or even vegetarian. Flexitarian (those that reduce meat consumption) or Pescatarian (forego meat and poultry but still consume fish and seafood products) are both plant-based eating patterns.

Being vegan is more than what you eat. It is a lifestyle choice. You will not only exclude, where possible, all food and drinks associated with the cruelty or exploitation of animals but other items, such as clothing. The vegan philosophy promotes the use of alternatives to help animals, humans, and the environment alike.

Vegan Is Not Always Healthy

The availability of vegan products has never been greater, and an exponential increase is expected between

2020 and 2025. But a large proportion of these products are heavily processed. Beneficial nutrients are stripped away during manufacturing, replaced by added sugars, salt, and saturated fats. All these additives can increase the risk of cardiovascular disease, cancer, and high blood pressure.

Health professionals recommend a diet that contains fruits, vegetables, pulses, and grains, all of which have very little processing and can maximise your wellbeing. Compare this to chips, crisps, and cereals, technically free of animal products but far from nutritious.

Plant-Based Is Nutritious

You can get all the nutrients your body needs without eating meat, but iron deficiency is possible when following a plant-based plan. Meat products allow easier absorption of iron, but in conjunction with healthy amounts of Vitamin C, plant-based iron will achieve the required levels.

Most foods you eat provide the necessary vitamins and minerals, either through natural means or by fortification. Supplements for both B12 and iron may be required if you follow a strict plant-based plan. These are readily available in fortified plant-derived foods, including milk and cereals.

Plant-Based Provides Protein

If you are eating a healthy, varied, and balanced diet, you will be getting enough protein. With most people consuming significantly more protein than is required to function effectively, moving to a plant-based eating plan would still provide sufficient levels. If you are worried about getting adequate protein, increase your portion sizes. Making yourself fuller quicker reduces the risk of snacking. Try adding protein powders to your meals as another alternative.

Plant-Based Can Form Complete Proteins

Some essential amino acids are limited in plant protein sources. But you don't have to worry. Your body can form complete proteins from several sources consumed during different meals. If you follow dietary guidelines, your body has all the amino acids required to make all the new proteins it needs.

Plant-Based Is Suitable For Children

As a child, you may have turned your nose up at many vegetables, a natural reaction to the unknown. Your parents' response would be, *'How do you know you don't like it if you haven't tried it?'* Like adults, children need a nutritionally balanced healthy diet that provides the variety of vitamins and minerals required to develop and grow.

You can get the kids involved in selecting and preparing meals, using colours to introduce new fruits and vegetables. Create recognisable dishes with a plant-based origin, such as *Buffalo Cauliflower Wings* or lentil-based *Meatballs*, to make them feel comfortable with new choices.

If you are concerned about missing nutrients, such as B12, iron, calcium, or zinc, they can be introduced through approved supplements, making plant-based eating an option for the whole family.

Plant-Based Is Not Limited

Gone are the days where the only plant-based options were a salad, beans, and tofu. Choices are now limitless and wide-ranging in taste profile, with plant-based alternatives for all your favourite foods. Committing to eating more fruit, vegetables, legumes, and grain opens your palate to new flavours, ensuring you get those all-important nutrients.

Plant-Based Can Provide Calcium

With calcium forming the basis of strong bones, you need to absorb adequate levels. Surprisingly leafy greens, such as kale, cabbage, or Pak Choi, are more potent calcium sources than cow's milk. So, moving to a more plant-based eating pattern will not be detrimental to either bone strength or repair. Drink calcium-fortified fruit juices or plant-derived dairy to help keep levels high, and get outside as Vitamin D can help improve calcium absorption.

Cancer Risk Linked To Soy

A staple for East Asians for centuries, the soybean is a rich protein source and is traditionally found in foods such as tofu, tempeh, edamame, and miso. While there have been links to increased cancer risks, there is also conjecture that soy can reduce the chance of developing it. There have also been links to soy reducing the risk of heart disease and possibly cholesterol.

REFLECTION

Keep a food diary for the next seven days, and then answer these questions.

1. **How many portions of fruit or vegetables do you eat a week?**

2. **What proportion of your diet comes from the five main food groups?**

3. **What actions could you take to improve the balance in your diet?**

11. POWER YOUR FITNESS

It's January. *New Year, New Me.* Again.

Every year you set off with the intention of improving your fitness or health, and by the middle of February, you are back at square one. Why does it keep happening?

Racing headlong into the latest exercise fad, seeking out quick results is one of the biggest reasons. You make no consideration for your underlying fitness, the time you have available, or whether you will enjoy the activity. Combining this with setting weight loss goals, rather than concentrating on how it makes you feel, is not a recipe for success.

With any change, you must, first and foremost, want to make it. But coming a very close second is a positive environment. One that makes the process enjoyable, producing successful and sustainable methods and results in the process.

Exercise and training should make you feel good. It releases endorphins, increases energy, and gives you positive vibes, allowing a virtuous circle to form around your fitness plans. You can often underestimate these simple benefits, and be aware, as there is one thing that can derail them.

THE MOOD HOOVER

You will all know a *mood hoover*. It's that pessimistic and critical person who rapidly drains the positive energy out of any situation. They may even be friends or family members, making it a tad awkward if you want to take action, as their thoughts can be far from constructive. Try to unplug yourself by limiting your time with them, developing positive energy in and around your support bubble in the process. The environment you create must allow you to project and receive positive feelings about your fitness goals. Emotions are contagious, and optimistic outpourings can go a long way in delivering impressive results.

The Mood Hoover principle is not just about people. It can apply to material items, with mobile phones, television, and other media feeding a constant barrage of *newsworthy* negativity. At every opportunity draining our positivity and energy. But the worst of them all is lurking in the bathroom, the dreaded set of weighing scales.

By constantly jumping on the scales, you can quickly kill the motivation required to get, and stay, fit. You may have experienced this feeling, working hard in the gym, sweating like no tomorrow, but jumping on the scales tells a different story. No weight loss, which feels deflating, the negative thought of '*what's the point*?' begins to manifest. It can be the same if you follow weight loss programmes. Stick to the rules all week, feel fantastic, and then weigh-in Wednesday arrives. You see no change or worse, an increase. You start dreading every *hump day*, and the same '*what's the point?*' feeling starts to rise.

Weighing scales take no account of the softer metrics that come with healthy eating and fitness. How your body composition changes, the increased energy, and the improvement in underlying fitness and strength. Completing a session makes you feel satisfied and sets happy hormones racing around your body. Your happiness and confidence all come from feeling good. Simply put, the scales don't measure sexy.

FAT VERSUS LEAN MUSCLE

Excessive body fat contributes to significant health risks, including heart attacks, strokes, and high blood pressure. By combining a healthier diet, with increased exercise, you can start burning this fat and, in the process, build lean muscle. This newly formed muscle tissue is denser than fat, meaning your body composition influences your weight. Being more athletic and healthier may lead to you appearing thinner than someone of the same height and weight—another challenge of using scales to judge your health.

Body Mass Index (BMI)

BMI is a standard medical term used to measure health, with a value of between 19 and 25 being considered healthy. But as a by-product of two numerical measurements, your height and weight, there is no consideration of body shape, composition, or physical and mental fitness levels. To illustrate the point, consider these generic but realistic statistics.

A Defensive End in the National Football League may stand at six feet five inches, weigh in at a muscular 290 pounds and run 40 yards in less than five seconds. His BMI works out at 34, putting him at the top of the obese range.

An international Rugby Union back-row forward could stand at six feet two inches tall and weigh 280 pounds. Their BMI is an even 'unhealthier' 36.

Nobody who has watched these sports, with these players operating at the peak of their powers, can say they look unhealthy and certainly not overweight.

It means that a holistic approach is required when measuring your health and fitness and start by removing the weighing scales. Taking them away may be a daunting prospect. You may have been using them habitually for years, but it is time to kick the habit. If you are a serial weigh-in king or queen, start by taking a day off, weigh in alternate days, and track your four-weight average. You are more likely to observe consistent progress, removing any negative influence a single weigh-in can have.

By considering how you monitor progress, you are more likely to keep momentum and enjoy positive results. Try one, or more, of the following options as an alternative method of tracking results.

Progress Pictures

These provide a great reminder of success if your motivation wanes and are a consistent way to track your progress over time. Photos are much better than using real-time methods, such as scales or a mirror. Both of these can create mental barriers, with your mind playing tricks that may hamper your results.

The Good Old-Fashioned Tape Measure

Tracking your natural waist indicates the level of abdominal fat you are carrying. Understanding this is important as it links directly to the risk of suffering heart disease and other medical conditions.

The measurement is taken around your torso, just above the belly button, and gives an effective alternative to BMI. A waist circumference of 35 inches or more in women and 40 inches or more for men places you at increased risk of developing cardiovascular problems.

By taking a second measurement, this time from your hips' broadest part, you can calculate your waist-to-hip ratio by dividing your waist circumference by your hip circumference. Results above 0.90 for males and above 0.85 for females represent abdominal obesity.

Body Fat Measuring

The simplest way to calculate your body fat is by using a specially designed calliper. Often used by medical professionals, they are readily available and reasonably priced for you to purchase. Skin and fat measurements from the waist, shoulder blade, biceps, and triceps, are combined into a single measure, with the result plotted against your age and sex to determine your body fat percentage. The higher the value, the higher your risk of suffering from obesity-related conditions.

Remember, how you feel is as, if not more, important than any numerical measurement, and your ideal weight is whatever you reach when you live the healthiest life you enjoy.

WHAT IS FITNESS?

Fitness is the measure of the body's ability to function efficiently and effectively in work and leisure activities. And being fit might have a different meaning for every person. It may be a personal achievement, such as climbing Kilimanjaro or running a marathon, or it can simply be not being out of breath when climbing the stairs. Whatever the aim or goal, make it personal to you and consider the next section's ideas to help you achieve them.

A DIFFERENT APPROACH

The modern world is demanding on your time, money, and health. With new habits take time to form, your fitness regimes will be no different. Until they embed in your routines, the results you desire can be challenging to deliver. In a world where looking perfect is deemed more important than how you feel, it is easy to focus on short-term gains rather than long-term change. To make your goals personal, realistic, and achievable, consider the following three suggestions.

It's A Marathon, Not A Sprint

What's the rush? You've got the rest of your life to get fit and stay fit. Estimates suggest that 80% of New Year's resolutions are broken within six weeks, not even making it past the middle of February. The reason, the world is fast-paced, and you believe your fitness improvements should be too.

Take your time to find what works for you, the best time to train, and the type of exercise. Gradually increasing frequency and intensity reduces the risk of injury and builds a regime that is likely to stick. And listen to your body. If it is telling you to rest, then rest. If you are feeling energised, then run that extra kilometre or smash out another 20 burpees.

Do Something You Love

If you don't enjoy how you keep fit, you are less likely to stay on the path to sustainable change. The mind and body prefer pleasure to pain, so you need to create a positive feeling about training and the challenges it brings. Making exercise attractive holds your attention span better, and you will start to embrace a no pain no gain philosophy. And if you love the result, like anything in life, you want to repeat it. The endorphin rush becomes addictive in a good way, and you will thrive on this feeling.

You could also get creative, trying different activities at different times of the day. If you struggle to get up early to run, drag yourself to the gym or smash out a HIIT session, then try sessions in the evening or over lunch if you have the flexibility. A lunchtime walk or run, a high-intensity workout in the local park, even cycling to work introduces variation to make fitness more enjoyable. Give yourself permission to make mistakes and take the time to get it right.

Getting Into A Rhythm

Although they are fun and energetic, this section isn't about taking a Zumba or Salsa class. A simple approach to successful fitness is finding a rhythmic pattern around when you exercise. You know from earlier chapters that the brain loves structure and patterns, so why not use them to formulate exercise regimes.

You could train on the same days every week or try three consecutive days followed by a rest day. It may require some trial and error, but with time you will discover what works for you. And do remember to take your time. Going all guns blazing seven days a week increases the risk of injury, which can knock your confidence, slowing or even stopping momentum before you have even got started.

TYPES OF ACTIVITY

There are four main types of exercise: *cardiovascular, resistance, balance, and flexibility*, and varying between them is essential to delivering sustainable results. The apathy of repeating the same form of training can often lead to you stopping exercise altogether. By exercising different parts of the body in varied ways, you can also prevent injuries from occurring. Think about the approach a bodybuilder takes to training, with a leg day, followed by chest and then arms. No muscle groups are exercised on consecutive days.

The different types of exercise are not mutually exclusive either and often complement each other. As an example, resistance training builds muscle, which improves your balance and posture. You can then exercise for longer and increase cardiovascular endurance in the process.

Let's explore how to get the best out of the four types of exercise.

Cardiovascular

These activities are aerobic or endurance-based, aimed at increasing your breathing and heart rate. Helping you perform everyday tasks more effectively and efficiently they keep you healthy and improve general fitness. It is important to focus specifically on your heart, lungs, and cardiovascular systems, as improving your health in these areas prevents the onset of diseases that develop with age (e.g., diabetes, colon and breast cancers, and heart disease).

You don't have to run for miles either. A brisk walk, dancing, or swimming will provide fantastic health benefits. Even mowing the lawn or climbing the stairs, tasks you maybe take for granted, count as aerobic exercise. As your staying power improves, you can progress to climbing mountains and running marathons if you choose to. You can quite literally *walk before you can run* when improving your fitness.

Whether you are starting from scratch or returning to training after an enforced layoff, seek advice from your doctor. Start slowly, listen to your body, and avoid overexertion from the outset. Cardiovascular activities should not make you feel dizzy or cause chest pain or pressure. Immediately stop exercising if you exhibit any of these symptoms, and consider seeking medical advice.

Your aim could be to build up to two to three hours a week of exercise that makes you breathe hard. To test the intensity of your training, try talking while being active. If you can hold a conversation but are breathing hard, then it is considered moderate intensity. Once you begin taking a breath after every few words, then you have hit high intensity.

As you have already discovered, be creative to keep it interesting, and there are imaginative ways to stay active during the day. If your job is not physical, then consciously take time to walk around, take the stairs instead of the lift, or park further from the office to increase your steps. Try to remain active throughout your day and avoid sitting for long periods.

If your training activity is more strenuous, then complete both a warm-up and cool-down session. A small number of stretches before, during, or after your workout can make all the difference. It doesn't matter whether you are jogging or sweeping the drive; you will use muscles that you don't typically. They will be shocked into action and react if you don't pre-warn them with stretches. You can explore stretching later in the chapter, and Appendix II shares some basic exercises you can try.

It is essential to stay hydrated during any physical activity, and especially cardiovascular exercise. Make sure you drink water regularly, replenishing the electrolytes lost through sweating (see more about hydration in chapter nine). Water provides all the essential nutrients you need to replace, so there is not always a need for fancy isotonic drinks either. There is more about the pros and cons of these types of drinks later in the chapter.

Finally, when exercising outdoors, be aware of the environment around you. Watch out for vehicles if running on the street, have enough ambient lighting to avoid trips and slips, and exercise in an area you know well. Consider the temperature and type of activity when choosing the appropriate clothing. Wear layers in colder weather, grab that bicycle helmet when cycling, or strong walking boots if hiking. Safety is hugely important during all types of training.

Resistance

Often referred to as strength training, improving your stability through resistance activities can be hugely beneficial. Strong muscles make everyday tasks, such as climbing the stairs or carrying the shopping, much more manageable. Plus, there will be no funny noises when bending down or rising from the sofa.

Routine resistance exercises include lifting weights, using resistance bands, and swimming. These exercises help you form a stable core, improving balance and reduce the risks of falls.

In chapter six, you read how vital breathing correctly can be, and in the case of resistance training, it allows you to perform exercises effectively and efficiently. Take slow and steady breaths, exhaling as you lift or push, and then inhaling as you relax. Never hold your breath during resistance training, as it adds further pressure to the blood flow, increasing it to an uncomfortable and potentially dangerous level.

<u>Weight Training</u>

Remember that your body needs to adapt to resistance training. Don't be concerned or embarrassed if you start using two-kilogram dumbbells or kettlebells. Nobody likes a show-off and overexerting not only increases the risk of injury but can also affect form, meaning you may complete exercises ineffectively. You should make smooth, steady moves, avoid swinging weights into position, and don't lock out your arms or legs. If you are using strength training regularly, avoid exercising the same major muscle groups on consecutive days.

Investing in a gym membership will give you access to fantastic equipment, but you can get equally good results at home. There is reasonably priced equipment available online, and you can even use everyday household items. Bottled water or tinned foods make great dumbbells, and bags of flour can substitute kettlebells. Perhaps consider this as a way to build up fundamental strength before braving the gym.

Resistance Bands

Try replacing weights with these large elastic bands. With various resistance levels, you develop strength as you progress, steadily become more comfortable with the exercises. You can combine different bands to form new tension levels, and as with weights, slow and steady is the order of the day. With most bands having handles, this helps avoid slips and injuries.

Balance

These exercises improve your stability when performing other types of training. Lower body exercises, such as lunges or squats, Yoga, and Tai Chi, aim to strengthen the core and straighten posture. Both Yoga and Tai Chi are based on age-old principles of slow, gentle, and precise body movements while breathing deeply. Refer back to chapter six (Power Your Breathing) for some basic poses and transitions.

You can try these simple balance exercises, all in the comfort of your own home.

See how long you can stand on one foot, and then swap.

Get out of your chair without using your hands or arms for support.

Walk using the heel-to-toe technique, putting the heel of your right foot in front of the toes of your left foot, alternating as you walk between rooms.

Flexibility

By stretching regularly, your flexibility can improve dramatically, making movement easier in all other activities. You find it easier to bend down, pick up the kid's toys, or tie your shoes. And looking over the shoulder becomes so much easier. As well as helping balance, Tai Chi and Yoga are also great activities to improve your flexibility.

While stretching can be an individual activity, consider including it before and after cardiovascular or strength training. It aids muscle recovery, releases lactic acid, and helps avoid injury. When completing flexibility routines, you should breathe normally and avoid overstretching. You hit the sweet spot when suffering a little discomfort as you stretch.

DOMS

Whether you have heard of it or not, you can never mistake it. Anyone who has gone back to training or taken it up for the first time will have experienced the torture of *DOMS*. It's the one thing nobody tells you about when you decide to get fit. You hear about all the fantastic transformations your body will go through, but less about the pain.

DOMS, or *Delayed-Onset Muscle Soreness* to give its full title, is like a fitness ninja. It jumps out, taking you by surprise one or two days after a workout. You may struggle to bend down or negotiate the stairs, muscles aching throughout the body.

The good news is you are not alone, and even professional athletes suffer the torture of DOMS. You should see it as a positive sign. You are doing something right, although you may need to embrace pain for a while.

When you suffer from DOMS, there is a preconception that it's due to a lack of oxygen in the body, leaving it struggling to break down glucose, which results in a lactic acid build-up in the muscles. The actual reason is a temporary inflammation around the muscles, resulting in blood cells rushing to repair the micro-tears caused by the training.

DOMS is a perfectly normal feeling, with your muscles building back more robust and firmer as your body starts to transform. After around 48 hours, you will be well on the way to recovery, and there are several ways to alleviate the symptoms during this time.

Continue To Exercise

Given the potential pain, this is probably not your first choice, but low-impact cardio, such as walking or swimming, is a great option. Practicing Yoga, Pilates, or simple stretches will also reduce the soreness.

Temperature Applications

Professional athletes use ice baths to combat the inflammation caused by the micro-tears in the muscles. Not the most appealing of ideas, but you can replicate the process at home by sitting in a cold bath. If that is not your thing, then there is a warmer option. Grab a cup of Epsom salts and drop it into a hot bath. The magnesium it contains helps widen the blood vessels, aiding recovery by soaking the soreness away. You can contrast the therapy, alternating between hot and cold for around 10 to 20 minutes. Try swapping between a warm bath and cold shower, or interchange hot and cold compresses for specific muscle groups.

Foam Rollers

A great addition to your fitness equipment is a foam roller. By slowly rolling each major muscle group, you can release tightness and knotting in the muscle fibres. Make the treatment more effective by deep breathing and changing the angles to target more profound tears.

Compression Garments

It is a regular occurrence to see elite athletes wearing knee-high compression socks before, during, and after an event. They can help in the following three areas and ease the recovery from DOMS in the process.

Circulation

During exercise, your muscles act as subsidiary pumps, helping the heart drive blood through the body. By wearing graduated compression garments that tighten at the extremities, you can increase this blood flow further. As you train, waste products are removed from the body more efficiently, providing more oxygen to the muscles and reducing potential swelling.

Lymph Drainage

The lymph vessels control the process of removing excess fluids and waste from cells. The compression garments improve the efficiency of this function, speeding up recovery and healing.

Muscle Protection

By reducing the impact on muscles, the compression garments reduce inflammation, swelling, and muscle damage caused by exercise.

One note of caution is that you should not overuse compression garments or wear them incorrectly, as this may cause more problems than solve. Risks include broken skin and possible infections.

STRETCHING

Adding regular stretching to your routine prevents injury, aids recovery, and reduces the impact of *DOMS*. For these reasons, it holds equal importance as the actual exercise or activity in keeping you healthy.

Before exercise, stretching increases your body's flexibility. The more pliable your major muscle groups are, the less likely you are to sustain an injury. The stretches you perform should target those muscles that you plan to exercise. For example, if you are going for a run, focus on stretching your hamstrings, quads, glutes, and calves, holding each stretch for 10 to 20 seconds.

Post-workout stretches are great at removing excess lactic acid from the body, freeing up movement, and resetting the muscles to their original length. Target those major muscle groups used during the workout to reduce the tension and relax the muscles. Try holding your post-workout stretches for a little longer, perhaps 20 to 30 seconds, with Appendix II contains some great examples for you to try before and after exercise.

Stretching that can be completed independently of your regular training routine is also recommended. You may consider Yoga, an activity that can be practiced by everyone regardless of experience. The poses work on stretching your muscles, increasing flexibility, and reducing stiffness. After only eight weeks of practise, you could find your flexibility has improved by up to 35%.

Some Yoga styles are more physical by design and target muscle tone improvements, with less vigorous poses concentrating on strength and endurance, building core abdominal stability in most cases. Poses such as Downward Dog, Cobra (or Upward Dog), and the Plank develop your upper body strength. Standing poses such as the Warrior, Triangle, or Tree build your hamstrings, quads, and glutes.

ISOTONIC DRINKS

Hydration is back on the agenda as you close out this chapter. If you watch sport regularly, you will have seen athletes grabbing an isotonic drink to replenish their fluids. These drinks are full of the vitamins and nutrients that are lost during the match or event.

While they are seemingly essential for elite athletes, in most cases, water provides all the necessary nutrients you need after a training session.

So, do you even need isotonic drinks?

Let's take a look at the pros and cons.

Advantages

<u>Replacing Fluids</u>
Sweating occurs when you exercise, removing essential fluids and vitamins that help the body function effectively. For this reason, elite athletes and highly active adults grab that sports drink after a training session or match.

<u>It is not Water</u>
Although water can be the best thing to drink after training, it is good to vary your fluid intake. Sports drinks provide that change and an alternative for those who don't enjoy drinking water.

<u>Carbohydrates & Protein</u>
By introducing carbohydrates into your body quickly, isotonic sports drinks can energise muscles, ensuring they operate effectively and efficiently. Some products choose to couple protein with carbohydrates, which may improve your performance further.

<u>Digestion</u>
Fluids are more straightforward to digest than food, and if your body is feeling anxious or under pressure, processing solids can be affected. The drinks' vitamins and minerals help the body feel full and digest those essential elements it needs to perform.

Disadvantages

<u>Acidity</u>
Isotonic drinks can be full of sugar and sodium, which can slowly dissolve the protective enamel on your teeth. When low on fluids, your body doesn't produce saliva efficiently. It is this saliva that removes potentially harmful substances from these drinks, thus protecting the teeth.

<u>Water Replacement</u>
It is only after at least 45 minutes of strenuous cardiovascular or aerobic activity that the increased concentration of vitamins and nutrients that sports drinks provide is warranted. Water provides sufficient fluid replacement for most average adults. For this reason, many organised marathons supply only water to the public participants.

<u>Sugar</u>
Excessive consumption of sugar can lead to diabetes, high blood pressure, and weight gain. With some sports drinks adding the equivalent of eight teaspoons of sugar, they can have a detrimental effect on your health if consumed in excess.

<u>Caffeine</u>
Caffeine is an ingredient in several sports drinks, with the equivalent of a canned soft drink or cup of coffee contained in some products. At these levels, it not only increases your energy levels but your blood pressure, which can potentially lead to other issues. Check out chapter eight (Power Your Detox) to find out more about caffeine's adverse effects.

REFLECTION

Consider how you can increase your exercise and improve your fitness.

1. **Which days and at what times are best for your exercise sessions?**

2. **How can you increase variety in the exercise you do?**

3. **How can you overcome the barriers stopping you from improving your fitness?**

12. POWER YOUR PLANNING

At some point in your life, you will have formulated a plan. It could be that fantastic summer holiday, a child's birthday party, or a project for work. You take the time to think about every activity or task needed to achieve the desired result. But, not only do you plan, you prepare. Mitigating risk, perhaps learning from previous outcomes, refining your plans to ensure success or happiness. You plan for the known and prepare for the unknown.

As an example, let's consider these two approaches to a family day trip.

Approach One
You decide to travel to the coast at the weekend, planning to enjoy a fun day at the beach. Saturday arrives, the sun is out, it's going to be a great trip. Everyone jumps into the car, and away you go. When you arrive at your destination, it is raining. Why, oh, why didn't you check the weather forecast? No coats, no changes of clothes, no fun at the beach.

Approach Two
Having decided to travel to the coast at the weekend, you start checking the weather forecast. Your preferred destination looks like it is going to be hit with rain all weekend. That's a no-go then, so an alternative location it is. Saturday looks like the best day, but there is a slight chance of rain in the afternoon. That's OK because you will set off early, enjoy some time at the beach, and then pop

over to the indoor activity centre you saw on the resort's website. Just in case, you pack a change of clothes. Everyone's happy, and you have a brilliant day out.

It is safe to say you will probably prefer to be on trip number two. You have mitigated some of the issues, making the day out as worry-free as possible.

How often do you apply this level of planning and preparation to your health and wellbeing?

You are most likely somewhere between the two examples, but to make real change in your life, you need to consider being almost military-like in delivering your desired outcomes. How many times have you promised to eat healthier, exercise more, or simply take better care of yourself? If the answer is more than once, then perhaps you need to consider a different approach.

Henry Ford once said, *if you always do what you always did, you always get what you always got*. Einstein defined insanity as *doing the same thing repeatedly and expecting different results*. You need to plan and prepare to create change in your lifestyle. Here are some ideas and techniques you can apply to deliver a healthier life.

FUELLING YOUR BODY

This section focuses on meal planning and preparation, but the principle of thinking about what you do and when and where you do it is adaptable for any area of fuelling your body. As you read through the section, consider how you could apply similar techniques to how you breathe, sleep and clear your mind.

You want to eat healthier, which is fantastic, but if you don't plan your meals, you are making it easier to pick up the phone for a takeaway or pop that ready meal in the microwave. When you take the time to plan where, when, and what you will eat, you are less likely to slip back into bad habits. Your preparation will improve as you know what ingredients and equipment you need to make these healthier meals.

Here are a few hints and tips that can help.

Plan When You Eat

You lead a busy life, and planning when you are going to eat, plus considering the length of time available, are essential for any healthy eating plan. You may want to go as far as putting mealtimes in your diary, as there is nothing more important than focusing on your health.

Plan What You Eat

Choose every meal for every day, selecting them based on when and how long you have to eat. Study your cookbooks, highlight and learn recipes and write everything down. You can even build healthy snacks and treats into your plan, just not too many. These straightforward actions will help you reduce poor nutritional choices during the week.

Write A Shopping List

How many times have you popped into the supermarket to get one thing then come away with yet another bag full of stuff you didn't want or need?

Writing a shopping list is a great way to focus on buying the right foods. You can even try taking it to the next level, visualising the supermarket layout, following the shelves' zig and zag, scribbling down your list as you go. You know your brain loves order, sequence, and patterns, and it will make the trip more efficient, and you will avoid dwelling around unhealthy food choices.

Preparing For Mealtime

It doesn't stop once the shopping trip is complete. Most people cite time, or not having it, as the reason not to eat healthily, so being efficient at mealtimes is paramount. You spend more time preparing and cooking food than eating it, and you will quickly realise there is plenty of time and easy ways to create more. Cook in larger quantities, and freeze or refrigerate batches for use later in the week. There are plenty of quick-cook recipe books on the market, providing healthy options in less than 30 minutes.

Get The Right Equipment

Any chef will tell you *buying cheap means buying twice*. You will be investing in your health by purchasing quality kitchen equipment, and you may be surprised to hear it won't break the bank. Here is a list of the essential items that make preparation easier:

Chef Knife Block (and sharpening tool)
Chopping Boards
Speed Peeler
Stick Blender
Mini Chopper
Food Processor
Oven Proof Sauté Pan
Large Casserole Pan

With these in the cupboard, you can rustle up any healthy meal.

Turn Your Kitchen Into A Cockpit

Get everything together before your start cooking. Set yourself up for success, with everything at arm's length, just like the cockpit of an aircraft. Use your space effectively and efficiently, with ingredients, recipes, and essential equipment ready to go. You will be amazed at how much easier it becomes to cook fresh nutritional food at home.

Make Convenience Foods Inconvenient

Convenience is a staple of the modern world, with takeaway and delivery never more accessible. Remove the numbers from your phone and then reflect on what you could cook in the 30-40 minutes it takes the delivery driver to arrive. Appendix I has some fantastic recipes if you are struggling, and only three are longer than 40 minutes.

FINDING FITNESS

Similar approaches can be applied to planning and preparing for the training sessions of your choice.

Plan Your Time

Go straight to your diary and block out the times you want to exercise. Don't compromise. It is your time, and nobody else can command your attention if you have reserved that time for a lunchtime stroll or an early morning gym session.

Choose Your Activity Wisely

You might love running, enjoy cycling, or be a HIIT fanatic. You may even throw a gym session in for good measure. Whatever your activity of choice, there are two considerations, making it enjoyable and timely. When you have planned training, choose a session that works for the time you set aside. There is nothing worse than cutting a session short, particularly one that you are enjoying.

Prepare Properly

Make sure you are stretching before, during, and after exercise. Look back at the previous chapter for why this is important, and perhaps use the stretches in Appendix II if you need inspiration.

But stretching is not the only preparation to consider. What if that 11:00 a.m. meeting overran? Can you push back the lunchtime walk? If not, what is the alternative? Focus on what you can control, and have a plan B. Often people don't train if they miss their time, and this can be a slippery slope. Two or three sessions fall by the wayside, and before you know it, you have fallen back into your previous bad habits. Remember, any exercise is better than no exercise.

Use The Right Equipment

Invest in your fitness, as you would with healthy eating. It may be a cushioned mat taking the strain off your joints, that perfect pair of trainers, or a lightweight kettlebell. Whatever it is, the correct equipment matters, and it can make all the difference to your results.

REFLECTION

1. **How can you improve your meal planning?**

2. **What action can you take to improve your exercise planning?**

3. **What kitchen or fitness equipment could you buy to help you become healthier?**

13. POWER YOUR RESULTS

This chapter starts with a gentle reminder.

YOU are the most important person.

You are the person who is in control but also need to hold yourself to account. Excellent results will follow if you deliver on those promises you made.

While other people may not act for you, they can help power your results and deliver those desired outcomes. If you choose wisely and surround yourself with the right people, you can create a support team, that group of individuals who understand what you are trying to achieve. By providing support, encouragement, and challenge at the correct times, they will keep you on track.

These are often known as:

ACCOUNTABILITY GROUPS

Why have an accountability group in the first place?

It is imperative to start with the end in mind, and sometimes your goal doesn't align with family members, friends, or peers. In this situation, an accountability group can be the solution.

Accountability groups can achieve so much by creating a haven with no judgement and providing the opportunity to share your highs and lows. They offer a supportive environment where problems are shared, helping you find solutions at times of challenge. Having the chance to assist other group members makes you feel happier, healthier and increases your positivity. It is as much about what you put in as what you get out.

What groups already exist?

There may be local or online groups already formed, so take the time to do your research. It is much easier joining an established group than starting your own from scratch. For example, you will find numerous health consultants holding weekly meetings, or you could create competition by synchronising your fitness app with fellow walkers, runners, or cyclists. Putting the research in at the beginning will reap massive rewards in the long term. Your accountability group may already be there. Find it, and more importantly, use it.

Who are the right people?

Firstly, talk to people who are committed to similar goals to you. They may be a good fit and are more than likely happy to discuss the idea and offer advice, but with no obligation to be involved.

Some of the best accountability groups are thrown together, started randomly, small groups within larger social communities. Having this mix of experience or personalities can create a more challenging environment but more satisfying results, so don't discount any approach to developing your group. It is about getting the right individuals who will exhibit these three key characteristics;

Trust

You have to trust all members, with no conversations leaked outside of the group. People, including you, may share personal feelings and thoughts, and the group must respect them.

<u>Open And Honest</u>
Becoming adept at giving and receiving feedback means being open and honest. Tough love, now and again, is no bad thing.

<u>Sociable</u>
The group will be spending regular time together, so surround yourself with people whose opinions you find exciting and insightful, prompting a social but challenging environment.

How many people does your group need?

That's up to you. There is no right or wrong answer, but here are some things to consider;

1. A face-to-face meeting is more manageable with fewer people (even more so virtually), but an online community or WhatsApp works well with a larger group.
2. The group is for everyone, so you need to make sure everyone gets their opportunity to share.
3. But not everyone needs to share at every meeting, so having help and support accessible when needed is essential.

What else should you consider?

Everyone is on an equal footing, so there are no mentoring relationships required, but you may find someone in the group more experienced or knowledgeable about a subject. Draw on them to help, but try and avoid asking them to provide the answer. If you arrive at a decision or agree to take action under your own steam, you are more likely to follow it through.

How you keep in contact can be crucial to success, so consider different mediums while ensuring it is frequent enough to avoid forgetting what you committed to at the previous session. You may choose instant messaging services (e.g., Slack, WhatsApp, and Messenger) that allow instant Q&A within the group or virtual catch-ups on Zoom, Teams, or Skype when geography or personal commitments are a challenge. And of course, you could meet in person. The choices are endless.

While the accountability group is there to help, often you find the more you put in, the more you get out. As you listen to others, something may trigger an answer to one of your challenges. But don't worry if you can't give an answer or provide advice. It is not a requirement to help everyone with everything. If you're unsure or don't know, be open and honest. Your accountability buddies will be grateful.

By vocalising your problem or challenge, and through the subsequent discussion, the answer often materialises. You can then set your goals and actions, and your accountability starts. Once you have set your targets, share them, and get ready to report back on them. When you have been successful, celebrate the wins, however big or small. All progress is good progress, and remember, sustainable change takes time to embed.

Even when you have achieved your goals, the benefits of the accountability group don't stop. Share challenges or problems you experienced along the way, discussing how you may have approached it differently. Always aim to achieve better results as effectively and efficiently as possible. A fantastic way to do this is to rate your progress out of ten and then ask, *'What could you improve to make it ten out of ten?'* It's a great discussion starter and a perfect way to get continual and consistent improvement.

What are some of the common pitfalls?

The first one is time creep. You've taken the time to find those like-minded people, the three or four fellow gym-goers, or members of your healthy eating programme. They are a great bunch. You get on like a house on fire and realise you have a lot more in common than you first envisaged. Don't lose focus. Consider setting some ground rules. You will be surprised how quickly time can get away from you.

The second is the dominator, a person who takes a disproportionate amount of time during the meeting. In some instances, if their challenge is sensitive or complex, it is warranted. But most of the time, it is ego taking over. Your meeting will be in danger of becoming a virtual or face-to-face marathon. Try nominating a chairperson for the group who can oversee timekeeping and facilitate free-flowing but timely conversation.

Overwhelm is another potential challenge. Everyone will start a new accountability group full of enthusiasm, charging in to support fellow members. This high-energy environment, driven by passion and bravado, can begin to be a little overwhelming at times. Imposter syndrome can kick in for some people, so remind yourself of the learning from chapter three (Power Your Imposter) if you find yourself in this situation. You may see it manifest through a lack of enthusiasm or showing disinterest in both sharing and contributing. It is more common than you think, and if you feel this way, don't beat yourself up about it. Be open with the group, share your thoughts, as there may be others feeling the same way.

What if you can't find a suitable accountability group?

Firstly, don't worry. Once you have set your goals and targets, start sharing your progress. You might post photos on Instagram, share recipe videos on Facebook or tweet your training programme for the week. It is an easy way to commit, deliver and keep yourself accountable for your actions.

You will find that once you've shared it and people have seen it, they start commenting and asking about your progress. It is a great feeling when someone checks in on you or gives you some fantastic feedback about your results. It creates a positive environment that keeps you accountable, generates momentum, and delivers sustainable change.

Get your partner or family members involved too. If they know your goals, they will probably ask about them every day. Have your progress update ready and impress them with how far you have come. They will also remind you about what you committed to, and more importantly, give you the kick up the backside you need to get back on track. Everyone needs little encouragement from time to time.

Sharing your goals gives you more clarity on what, how, and when you can achieve them. They become more realistic as you reflect on the feedback you receive. For instance, if you told a friend you will lose three stones in 30 days, they may look a little quizzical and question how healthy your approach will be. You may reflect on this, adjusting your goal to two or three pounds a week. A realistic and achievable target that makes it more likely you maintain a healthy weight.

What else can you do to deliver excellent results?

Teach. It is a great way to learn, form new habits, and deliver results. It even has a name.

THE PROTÉGÉ EFFECT

Proven to create a better understanding of a new subject and deliver better results, the Protégé Effect is a straightforward principle. It's an extension of the peer learning concept that you may have experienced at school or work. The central premise is that if you are going to teach something, you prepare better. You make sense of new material by mentally rearranging the information and merging it with what you already know. Combining this with teaching develops the long-term ability to retain, learn, and commit to the information or task.

Although it is not commonplace, this technique can be equally beneficial in your personal life. By considering the same approach to achieving a sustainable, healthier lifestyle, think how more effective you could be in getting results. You could try teaching the kids about the nutritional benefits of fruit and vegetables or your night owl friend about the benefits of high-quality sleep and, in the process, improve your understanding. As your knowledge grows, so does your commitment and accountability. You understand the benefits from the action you are taking and drive better results in the process.

REFLECTION

To maximise your results, you need support, so who, what, and how?

1. **Who can you approach to be in an accountability group?**

2. **What groups already exist to help deliver your goals?**

3. **How could you share what you have learnt from reading this book?**

14. POWER YOUR PASSIONS

Everyone has a moment in time when their passion gets ignited by a rewarding hobby, activity, or cause. Often driven by your desire to succeed, or the energy created by an inspirational individual, you feel *Fired Up* and *Ready to Go*.

In 2008, Illinois State Senator Barack Obama was closing in on a landslide victory in the US Presidential Election. His Republican opponent, John McCain, could not stem the tide of energy, belief, and momentum behind the Democrats' campaign. The distinctive atmosphere of hope and trust had inspired a nation, with a true leader breaking down barriers and taking everyone along for the ride. Obama was a charismatic candidate who enthralled people worldwide, increasing global interest in the election.

There are two slogans that define Obama's campaign.

Yes We Can and **Fired Up, Ready To Go!**

Both can be applied to your everyday thinking and inspire you to make sustainable changes in your life. The story behind *Fired Up, Ready to Go* is an excellent example of how you can generate the energy to deliver significant results.

The story starts in a small town called Greenwood in South Carolina. After a long day campaigning in the rain, Obama arrived tired and wet. By his own admission, he didn't want to be there.

He entered the small building in the local park, the venue for his campaign rally. His mood didn't improve when he realised there were only 20 people inside, all looking damp and sleepy, perhaps not wanting to be there either.

But what happens next was inspiring.

As Obama walked around, shaking hands and meeting people, he heard a voice behind him cry out, *Fired Up*. Caught a little off guard, he had no time to recover before everyone repeated the mantra. *Fired Up,* they all shouted.

Ready to Go, the original voice responded. Then, as if an everyday occurrence, the group responded in kind. *Ready to Go,* they cried.

Edith Childs, a local politician with Greenwood Council and an officer of the local NAACP (National Association for the Advancement of Coloured People), was the driving force behind this act. Her talents didn't end there, as she was a practising nurse who decided to study criminal justice after retirement—eventually becoming, of all things, a private investigator.

Edith took the chant wherever she went. The response, always the same as those 20 Greenwood residents. Obama described how she continued chanting *Fired Up, Ready to Go*, and the more she did, the more he felt *Fired Up* and *Ready to Go*. It was infectious, and he and his team thrived off the energy.

It was so simple but had such a far-reaching impact. By generating this level of passion for your health, you can take action and deliver stunning results. By applying and adapting the book's techniques, you can create a positive environment and experiences you will thrive on.

Edith also worked tirelessly to help support vulnerable people, developing school programmes, and facilitating meals for the unemployed. She even helped underprivileged families secure school supplies. A true heroine and superstar of the community, she was driven not by what she was doing but why she was doing it.

By reminding yourself of why you want to change, you will develop a passion for the ideas, techniques, and practices you adopt. You will get consistent results and be more adept at fighting off that devil known as Imposter Syndrome, creating a stable foundation in the process.

Four years on from his visit to Greenwood, Obama spoke about it at a 2012 re-election rally, closing his speech with these powerful words.

'One voice can change a room, and if it can change a room, it can change a city, and if it can change a city, it can change a state, and if it can change a state, it can change a nation, and if it can change a nation, it can change the world.'

Be that person, change the world, change your life.

Are You Fired Up?
Are You Ready To Go?

15. FINAL THOUGHTS

This book empowers you to make sustainable lifestyle choices, take back control, and create new long-lasting habits. You are now armed with the knowledge, practical techniques, and straightforward ideas to make it happen.

You have learnt that fuelling your body is about how you think, breathe, and sleep as much as what you consume. That essential nutrition, combined with different exercise types and the habit loop, can help you consistently eat healthily and improve fitness. In turn, this renewed energy feeds your passion for the activities you love, enabling you to achieve fantastic results.

The questions at the end of each chapter are designed to make you think and to prompt action. If you followed the *Be Honest, Be Open and Be Reflective* approach, you will have arrived at the changes you want. But to make them sustainable, you need to revisit the three objectives from earlier in the book; *Be Excited, Be Present and Be Curious*. Remind yourself how they link the ideas, techniques, and tips.

Be Excited

You have the passion for change, so turn that into action you love. If you are Fired Up, you will find that winning feeling mesmerising and addictive. Be excited by change, allow yourself to feel comfortable being uncomfortable, and make your life better in the process.

Be Present
Whatever action you take, do it in the moment. Recognise that you need to be flexible and adaptable to the situation, and remember to be kind to yourself if you fall off the proverbial waggon. Remind yourself these are just bumps in the road and that change doesn't come overnight. It takes time. It's a marathon, not a sprint.

Be Curious
Always question what you are doing and the impact it is having on your life. Be curious about why you make certain decisions and whether they optimise your sleep, breathing, and general health. Ask why specific techniques work for you and how you can develop continuous improvement through planning and preparation to drive better results.

Having read this book, you now know WHY you want to change, but more importantly, also the WAY to change. It's now up to you to consider one final action—your next step.

The Easy Option
Knowing you want to change but don't commit to taking action.

The Wasted Option
You apply some of the techniques on an ad-hoc basis and then wonder why the results don't come.

The Ultimate Option
You embrace everything you have read and learnt, and in the process, unleash the power of a healthy life.

Are You Fuelled, Fit and Fired Up?

APPENDIX I: THE RECIPES

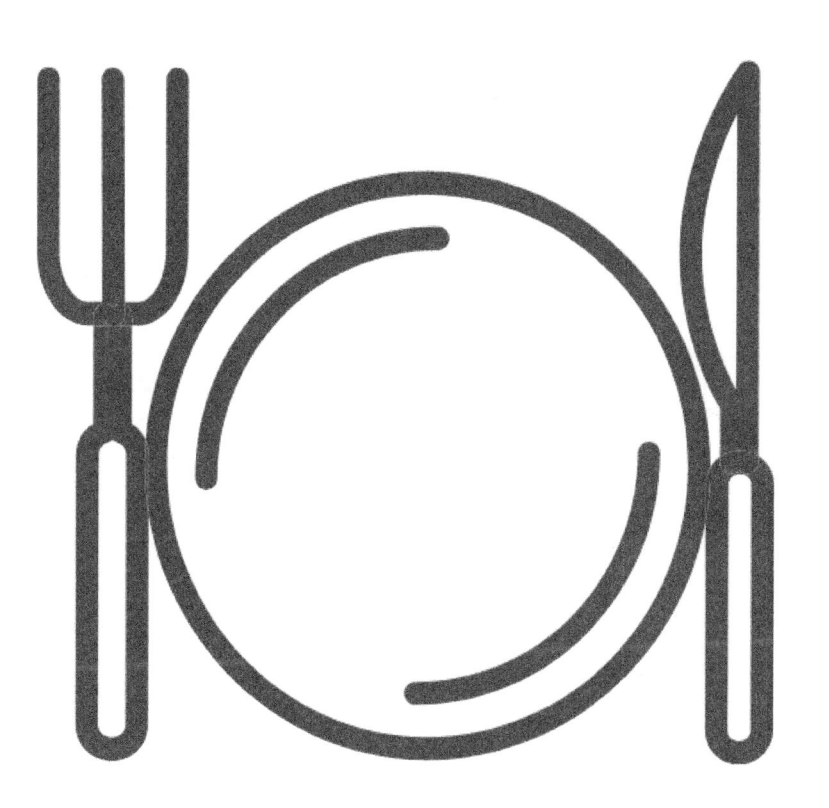

These are some of my favourite recipes, taking inspiration from Joe Wicks, The Boys from BOSH (Henry Firth & Ian Theasby), Jamie Oliver, The Hairy Bikers (Si King & Dave Myers), and Heather Thomas. A complete list of the books that inspired me is at the end of this appendix.

All of the recipes are meat-free, with the majority of ingredients being plant-based. There are some suggested ingredient swaps that you may enjoy, and you will be able to prepare all but three of the meals within 40 minutes.

Each meal spreads across two pages, with the first containing a brief description, the equipment you need, the ingredients, and the suggested swaps. The reverse page details the full recipe.

For those with a gluten or lactose intolerance, ingredients in *italics* can be swapped for suitable alternatives. For ease, the following key appears after the name of each dish:

V – VEGETARIAN

VE – VEGAN

GF – GLUTEN FREE OR GLUTEN FREE SWAP AVAILABLE

DF – DAIRY FREE OR DAIRY FREE SWAP AVAILABLE

If you do suffer from intolerances, then it is recommended you check the constituent ingredients of any sauces or prepared items to ensure they don't contain allergens.

CALIFORNIA SCRAMBLE (V, GF)

Estimated Time: 20 minutes

Serves: 2

This US-inspired brunch dish is the perfect start to a lazy Sunday morning. It is packed full of flavour, has a mild chilli kick, and is simple to cook.

Equipment:	**Ingredients:**
Jug	6 Eggs
Whisk	2 tbsp Olive Oil
Chopping Board	1 Red Chilli
Large Kitchen Knife	16 Cherry Tomatoes
Teaspoon	150g Baby Spinach
Tablespoon	100g Feta
Large Frying Pan	1 Avocado
Wooden Spoon	Salt
Kitchen Scales	Black Pepper

Mix It Up:

Try swapping the cherry tomatoes for a baby plum variety or add spring onions for extra flavour.

CALIFORNIA SCRAMBLE (V, GF)

Recipe:

1. Crack the eggs into a jug and whisk well, so the yolks and whites combine. Then season with a pinch of salt & black pepper.

2. Remove the stem from the chilli, deseed, and then finely chop. Halve the tomatoes. Halve and destone the avocado, scoop out the flesh with a teaspoon and finely slice.

3. Heat the oil in a large frying pan over medium heat. Throw in the chopped chilli and halved tomatoes, cooking for about 2 minutes until the tomatoes burst. Add the spinach and cook until wilted, and then pour in the eggs.

4. Turn the heat down to low and slowly scramble the eggs, bringing the cooked eggs from the edges into the middle of the pan.

5. Once cooked, tip onto a plate, sprinkle with the crumbled feta, and add the sliced avocado.

BREAKFAST HASH TACOS (VE, GF, DF)

Estimated Time: 20 minutes

Serves: 4

Vibrant, colourful, and inspired by Mexican cuisine, these tacos are brunch with a twist. Increase the heat with hot sauce or enjoy as they come.

Equipment:

Chopping Board
Large Kitchen Knife
2 Bowls (1 Microwaveable)
Clingfilm
Large Frying Pan
Wooden Spoon
Tablespoon
Teaspoon
Fine Grater
Kitchen Scales
Microwave

Ingredients:

1 Red Onion
3 tbsp Red Wine Vinegar
Salt
Sugar
200g New Potatoes
200g Chestnut Mushrooms
4 Plant-Based Sausages
2 tbsp Olive Oil
8 Corn Tortillas
1 Avocado
200g Cherry Tomatoes
4 Spring Onions
1 Garlic Clove
2 tsp Fajita Seasoning
100g Baby Spinach
30g Fresh Coriander

Mix It Up:

Swap the chestnut mushrooms for your own choice, and consider baby plum rather than cherry tomatoes. Add kale instead of the baby spinach for a little more crunch.

BREAKFAST HASH TACOS (VE, GF, DF)

Recipe:

1. Peel and finely slice the red onion. Add to the bowl with the red wine vinegar and a pinch of salt and sugar. Toss to combine and set aside for later.

2. Chop the potatoes into bite-size chunks. Put them into a microwaveable bowl, cover with clingfilm, and microwave on full power (800W) for 5 minutes until soft.

3. Meanwhile, slice the mushrooms and roughly chop the sausages. Put a frying pan on high heat and add the oil. Once hot, add the mushrooms and sausage, along with a pinch of salt. Fry for 5 minutes, stirring occasionally.

4. Halve and destone the avocado, scoop out the flesh with a teaspoon and finely slice. Halve the tomatoes and slice the spring onions.

5. Take the cooked potatoes and add them to the sausage and mushroom mix. Peel and grate in the garlic, sprinkle over the fajita seasoning, and cook for 2 minutes. Add the spinach and cook until wilted. Then add the tomatoes and spring onions.

6. Heat the tortillas in the microwave before evenly distributing the cooked hash between them. Top with pickled onion and sliced avocado.

CREAMED SPINACH WITH EGGS (V, GF, DF)

Estimated Time: 30 minutes

Serves: 4

A healthy version of Eggs Florentine, this tasty brunch provides a satisfying start to any day. It is surprisingly light on the calorie count, even with the cheese and single cream.

Equipment:

Chopping Board
Large Kitchen Knife
Large Frying Pan
Wooden Spoon
Teaspoon
Measuring Jug
Saucepan
Bowl
Tablespoon
Kitchen Scales

Ingredients:

10g Butter
1 Onion
¼ tsp Ground Cumin
½ tsp Ground Turmeric
Pinch of Cinnamon
Pinch of Nutmeg
300g Washed Spinach
150ml Single Cream
50g Grated Cheese
4 Eggs
Salt
Black Pepper

Mix It Up:

Try red onion or a small leek instead of the onion for a slight change in the flavour profile. You can also add texture by using kale rather than baby spinach

CREAMED SPINACH WITH EGGS (V, GF, DF)

Recipe:

1. Finely chop the onion while melting the butter in a large frying pan over medium heat. Add the onion to the pan with a pinch of salt, and cook for 6-8 minutes, until soft and translucent. Add the spices, along with some black pepper, and stir until they coat the onions thoroughly.

2. Roughly chop the spinach leaves and add them to the pan in batches. Stir until wilted before adding more spinach. Turn up the heat slightly and continue to cook for a further 5 minutes or until any liquid from the spinach has evaporated.

3. Pour in the cream, keep stirring until it has reduced, and then add half the grated cheese. Stir until the cheese has melted.

4. Bring a saucepan of water to the boil and add the eggs, boiling them for 6 minutes. Remove the eggs from the pan, placing them in a bowl of cold water to stop the cooking process. Carefully peel the eggs, cut in half, and then push the eggs into the spinach yolk side up.

5. Sprinkle over the remaining grated cheese, and then place the pan under a grill to melt the cheese and heat everything through.

ONE PAN BRUNCH (V, GF, DF)

Estimated Time: 25 minutes

Serves: 4

This Greek-inspired dish is colourful, mouth-watering, and enjoyable at any time of the day.

Equipment:

Chopping Board
Large Kitchen Knife
Garlic Press
Tablespoon
Large Frying Pan with Lid
Wooden Spoon
Teaspoon
Kitchen Scales

Ingredients:

2 tbsp Olive Oil
2 Red Onions
2 Garlic Cloves
1 Red Chilli
250g Halloumi
300g Baby Plum Tomatoes
500g Baby Spinach
4 Eggs
200g Greek Yoghurt
1 tsp Za'atar
A Handful of Fresh Parsley
Salt
Black Pepper
Hot Sauce

Mix It Up:

Don't worry if you haven't got Za'atar. Simply use ½ tsp Oregano and ½ tsp Thyme. The dish tastes equally good with white onion, and try cherry tomatoes alongside the baby plum variety.

ONE PAN BRUNCH (V, GF, DF)

Recipe:

1. Peel and finely chop the red onion. Peel and mince the garlic.

2. Remove the stem from the chilli, deseed and then dice.

3. Heat the oil in a large frying pan over medium heat. Cook the red onions, garlic, and chilli, for 6-8 minutes or until they soften, stirring occasionally.

4. Cube the halloumi and add to the pan, cooking for 3-4 minutes, stirring until it's golden brown and crusty

5. Halve the tomatoes, adding them to the pan, and mix well. Add the spinach in batches, stirring until wilted.

6. Season with a pinch of salt and black pepper.

7. Make four hollows in the mixture and break an egg into each one. Reduce the heat, cover the pan and cook until the whites set.

8. Place dollops of yoghurt between the eggs and dust with Za'atar. Chop the parsley and sprinkle over the top before serving with a slight drizzle of hot sauce.

SPRING ONION, SPINACH, AND CHEESE FRITTATA (V, GF, DF)

Estimated Time: 20 minutes

Serves: 2

A simple, quick, and super-fuelled start to the day, this frittata is one of the most flexible brunch dishes, so try experimenting with some other ingredients.

Equipment:

Tablespoon
Large Frying Pan
Chopping Board
Large Kitchen Knife
Teaspoon
Mixing Bowl
Whisk
Kitchen Scales

Ingredients:

6 Eggs
4 Spring Onions
150 – 200g Baby Spinach
100g Grated Cheese
½ tsp Chilli Flakes
2 tbsp Olive Oil
Salt
Black Pepper
20g Fresh Dill
20g Fresh Parsley
1 Avocado

Mix It Up:

Swap or add in other green herbs, such as coriander or basil, while adding some cherry tomatoes for colour. Finely chopped red onion can be used instead of the spring onion, and try some asparagus or tenderstem broccoli instead of the baby spinach.

SPRING ONION, SPINACH, AND CHEESE FRITTATA (V, GF, DF)

Recipe:

1. Heat the olive oil in a large frying pan over medium heat. Slice the spring onions, add them to the pan, and cook for 5 minutes until soft.

2. Finely chop the dill and parsley. Crack the eggs into a bowl and whisk together with the herbs, chilli flakes, and ¾ of the grated cheese. Then season with salt and black pepper.

3. Return to the frying pan, adding the baby spinach in batches, and cook until wilted. Pour in the mixture from the bowl and cook for 3-4 minutes until the bottom and sides are firm. Remove from the hob and place under the grill, at medium heat, until the eggs cook and rise slightly.

4. Halve and destone the avocado. Scoop out the flesh and finely slice. Serve with the frittata.

SPICY HALLOUMI BURGER AND SWEET POTATO FRIES (V, GF, DF)

Estimated Time: 25 minutes

Serves: 2

An excellent option for lunch, as it is flexible and easy to cook. You can also bulk it up with some side salad or even guacamole. Whatever you choose, this fantastic dish won't disappoint.

Equipment:

Chopping Board
Large Kitchen Knife
3 Mixing Bowls
(Small, Medium and Large)
Tablespoon
Teaspoon
Baking Tray
Baking Parchment
Bread Knife
Large Frying Pan
Kitchen Scales

Ingredients:

6 tbsp Peri-Peri Sauce
200g Halloumi
2 tbsp Mayonnaise
1 Baby Gem Lettuce
1 Beef Tomato
2 Brioche Buns
1 Large Sweet Potato
Salt
Black Pepper
1 tbsp Olive Oil
1 tsp Smoked Paprika

Mix It Up:

Bulk up the burger with a couple of slices of cucumber or red onion. Change the taste profile by swapping out the halloumi for pressed tofu, or try a chipotle or sweet chilli sauce for the marinade.

SPICY HALLOUMI BURGER AND SWEET POTATO FRIES (V, GF, DF)

Recipe:

1. Scrub the sweet potato and then cut it into fries, leaving the skin in place. Place them into the large mixing bowl with one tablespoon of olive oil, a sprinkle of salt and black pepper, and a teaspoon of smoked paprika. Toss together, so the fries are evenly covered, and then layout on the lined baking tray. Place in a preheated oven (220°C or 200°C fan assisted) for 20-25 minutes.

2. Cut the halloumi into eight thin slices. Pour two tablespoons of Peri-Peri sauce into a medium mixing bowl and add the halloumi. Make sure both sides of the halloumi are covered and set aside to marinade.

3. In a small mixing bowl, stir the remaining Peri-Peri into the mayo, and set aside.

4. Separate the lettuce leaves and cut the beef tomato into slices, ready to build your burger. Slice the brioche buns in half and toast the inside under a grill.

5. Warm a non-stick frying pan over high heat and dry fry the halloumi for two minutes on both sides. Then remove from the heat and set aside.

6. Take your toasted burger bun, and add your spicy mayo to both halves. Stack the halloumi, lettuce, and tomato and serve with your sweet potato fries.

PORTOBELLO MUSHROOM BURGER AND ROSEMARY FRIES (V, GF, DF)

Estimated Time: 35 minutes

Serves: 4

This dish has a natural rustic feel, with the portobello mushrooms and herbs creating a fantastic flavour.

Equipment:

Chopping Board
Large Kitchen Knife
Mixing Bowl
Teaspoon
2 x Baking Trays
Baking Parchment
Garlic Press
Tablespoon
Kitchen Foil
Bread Knife

Ingredients:

8 Portobello Mushrooms
4 Garlic Cloves
1½ tsp Dried Rosemary
1 tsp Dried Thyme
6 tsp Olive Oil
2 tsp Balsamic Vinegar
4 Brioche Buns
1 Tomato
1 Baby Gem Lettuce
½ Red Onion
4 tbsp Tomato Ketchup
4 tbsp Mayonnaise
Salt
Black Pepper
2 Large Potatoes

Mix It Up:

Add some zing to the mayonnaise by adding peri-peri or sweet chilli sauce. Lower the calorie count by either going 'naked' with no bun or swap in a seeded burger bun.

PORTOBELLO MUSHROOM BURGER AND ROSEMARY FRIES (V, GF, DF)

Recipe:

1. Wash and scrub the potatoes and then cut them into 1 cm slices. Cut each piece into 1 cm wide lengths. Place in a bowl with ½ teaspoon of rosemary and two teaspoons of olive oil. Season with salt and black pepper. Toss together, ensuring the fries are all covered. Place on a lined baking tray in a pre-heated oven (220°C or 200°C fan assisted) for 25-30 minutes.

2. Meanwhile, lay the mushrooms out on a flat surface with the stalks facing up. Peel and mince the garlic and spread it evenly across the mushrooms. Sprinkle the dried thyme and remaining rosemary over the mushrooms, and then drizzle each one with a bit of olive oil and balsamic vinegar. Then season with salt and black pepper.

3. Wrap each mushroom in a square of foil, placing them on a baking tray in the oven for 15 minutes.

4. Slice each brioche bun in half and toast them under a grill. Slice the tomato and wash and trim the gem lettuce. Slice the red onion. Then spread ketchup over the base and mayonnaise on the top of the burger buns.

5. Remove the mushrooms from the oven and place on the prepared burger buns (red onion, tomato, lettuce, and then the mushrooms). Serve on a plate alongside the fries.

BBQ SWEET POTATO QUESADILLAS (V, GF, DF)

Estimated Time: 20 minutes

Serves: 2

Mexico meets the Deep South with this action-packed lunch that bursts with flavour. The perfect dish for a sharer or a tapas-style buffet.

Equipment:

Peeler
Chopping Board
Large Kitchen Knife
Tablespoon
Microwaveable Bowl
Clingfilm
Mixing Bowl
Large Frying Pan
Sieve or Colander
Fork
Wooden Spoon

Ingredients:

2 Large Sweet Potatoes
1 Avocado
4 Spring Onions
Lime Juice
Salt
Black Pepper
1 tbsp Olive Oil
2 Garlic Cloves
400g Black Beans
2 tbsp Fajita Seasoning
4 Flour Tortillas
60g Grated Cheese
BBQ Sauce

Mix It Up:

Try using carrot or butternut squash instead of sweet potatoes, and add another twist with chickpeas instead of black beans. Season the mixture with your own choices to add some personalisation.

BBQ SWEET POTATO QUESADILLAS (V, GF, DF)

Recipe:
1. Scrub and peel the sweet potatoes and then cut them into 1 cm chunks. Place them in a microwaveable bowl with one tablespoon of water. Cover with clingfilm and then blast in the microwave for 8 minutes.
2. Halve and destone the avocado. Then scoop out the flesh and roughly mash in a bowl with a fork. Thinly slice the spring onions, including the green bits, and add half to the bowl. Add a good shot of lime juice, season with salt and black pepper, and then mix everything. Set aside the avocado dip for later.
3. Thinly slice the garlic and add it, along with the remaining spring onion and olive oil, to a large frying pan over medium heat. Drain and rinse the black beans using a sieve or colander and add them to the pan, along with the fajita seasoning. Stir and cook for another 2 minutes.
4. Tip the mixture into the bowl with the cooked sweet potato, and roughly mash everything together with a fork. Add a couple of tablespoons of lime juice, and season with salt and pepper.
5. Put the pan back on high heat, and place the first tortilla in the pan. Pile on the sweet potato and bean mix, add the grated cheese on top with a BBQ sauce drizzle. Top with the other tortilla and then cook for a minute or so on each side. Chop into pieces and serve with the avocado dip.

HUEVOS RANCHEROS (V, GF, DF)

Estimated Time: 20 minutes

Serves: 2

This traditional rural Mexican dish is packed full of flavour and is enjoyable at any time of the day.

Equipment:

Sieve or Colander
Tablespoon
Large Frying Pan
Wooden Spoon
Mixing Bowl
Chopping Board
Large Kitchen Knife
Bread Knife
Teaspoon

Ingredients:

2 tbsp Olive Oil
2 tbsp Chipotle Sauce
400g Black Beans
Salt
Black Pepper
Lime Juice
2 tbsp Dried Coriander
2 Eggs
2 Bagels
1 Avocado
100g Feta Cheese
Hot Sauce

Mix It Up:

Dry fry some halloumi instead of the feta, and add some spring onion for extra crunch. Chickpeas make a great alternative to black beans.

HUEVOS RANCHEROS (V, GF, DF)

Recipe:

1. Drain and rinse the black beans using a sieve or colander.

2. Heat half the oil in a frying pan over medium heat, add the chipotle paste and stir. Add the black beans with salt and black pepper, and use the back of your spoon to mash some of the beans. Once heated through, tip into a bowl, add the coriander and lime juice, and set aside.

3. Add the remaining oil to the pan and fry the eggs to your liking. Halve the bagels and toast the bagel under a grill (or in a toaster).

4. Meanwhile, halve and destone the avocado, scoop out the flesh and finely slice.

5. Assemble the completed dish, with the bagel covered in the black beans, topped with the sliced avocado. Lay the eggs on top, finishing it with crumbled feta and drizzle of hot sauce.

6. Finally, place the other half of the bagel on top.

ASPARAGUS, POTATO AND LEEK SOUP (VE, GF, DF)

Estimated Time: 35 minutes

Serves: 6

You cannot beat having a flavour-filled wholesome soup for lunch. This vegetable-based dish gives you lots of options when it comes to swaps, and if you want it to be a bit more rustic, then don't blitz it too much, and serve with some crusty bread.

Equipment:

Chopping Board
Large Kitchen Knife
Tablespoon
Large Casserole Pan
Wooden Spoon
Stick Blender

Ingredients:

1 tbsp Olive Oil
1kg Asparagus Spears
2 Large Baking Potatoes
3 Leeks
2 tbsp Dried Thyme
1.5l of Veg Stock

Mix It Up:

The great thing about soup is you can play around with the ingredients to your heart's content. Try broccoli or cabbage, instead of asparagus, or swap out the potatoes for swede. If you aren't a fan of leeks, use white or red onion, and don't be afraid to add extra herbs. Finally, try bulking it up with some parsnips, carrots, or butternut squash.

ASPARAGUS, POTATO AND LEEK SOUP (VE, GF, DF)

Recipe:

1. Heat the oil in a large casserole pan over medium heat.

2. Cut the asparagus into inch-long pieces and add to the pan.

3. Roughly chop the potatoes and leeks and add them to the pan.

4. Sprinkle in the thyme and stir well. Cover and leave to cook for around 15 minutes. Stir regularly to avoid bits sticking to the bottom of the pan.

5. Pour in the stock, bring to the boil and simmer for a further 15 minutes. Remove from the heat and then blitz with a stick blender until smooth, strain through a sieve and then season with salt and black pepper.

MUSHROOM CAESAR SALAD (VE, GF, DF)

Estimated Time: 35 minutes

Serves: 4

This vegan version of a mainstream classic salad is as flavoursome as the original. It is ideal for taking as a packed lunch or enjoying in the back garden with your barbecue.

Equipment:

Chopping Board
Large Kitchen Knife
3 Mixing Bowls
Tablespoon
2 Baking Trays
Baking Parchment
Wooden Spoon
Garlic Press

Ingredients:

400g Mixed Mushrooms
3 tbsp Olive Oil
2 tbsp Vegan Seasoning
300g Romaine Lettuce
Salt
Black Pepper
3 tbsp Nutritional Yeast
4 Slices of Brown Bread
1 tsp Mixed Herbs
½ tsp Garlic Powder
1 Garlic Clove
60g Dairy Free Mayo
1 tbsp White Wine Vinegar
Lemon Juice

Mix It Up:

Add a splash of colour with some cherry tomatoes and sliced radishes.

MUSHROOM CAESAR SALAD (VE, GF, DF)

Recipe:

1. Roughly chop the mushrooms into bite-size chunks. Put them in a bowl and drizzle with the olive oil, and sprinkle over the seasoning. Toss to combine. Add the mushrooms to a lined baking tray and roast in a preheated oven (200ºC or 180ºC fan assisted) for 25-30 minutes.

2. Cut the bread into cubes. Add the olive oil, herbs, garlic powder, and a pinch of salt and black pepper to a second bowl. Stir to combine, then add the bread and stir to cover the cubes evenly. Spread the cubes out on the second lined baking tray and bake for 15 minutes until crispy and golden.

3. While the mushrooms and bread are in the oven, start making the dressing. Peel and mince the garlic, putting it into the third mixing bowl along with two tablespoons of nutritional yeast, mayonnaise, and white wine vinegar. Add a couple of tablespoons of lemon juice and mix well. Season with salt and black pepper, taste, and add more lemon juice if required.

4. Trim and roughly chop the lettuce and lay it out on the plates. Add the croutons and then top with the roasted mushrooms. Finally, drizzle over the dressing and the remaining nutritional yeast.

RATATOUILLE RISOTTO (VE, GF, DF)

Estimated Time: 60 minutes

Serves: 4

This fantastic dish combines French and Italian cuisine, giving you a healthy and flavour-filled dinner option.

Equipment:

Chopping Board
Large Kitchen Knife
Baking Tray
Baking Parchment
Tablespoon
Saucepan
Large Frying Pan
Wooden Spoon
Garlic Press
Teaspoon
Ladle
Kitchen Scales
Measuring Jug

Ingredients:

1 Aubergine
1 Courgette
6 Tomatoes
4 tbsp Olive Oil
1 Red Onion
2 Garlic Cloves
5 Sundried Tomatoes in Oil
1 tsp Dried Rosemary
1 tsp Dried Thyme
900ml Vegetable Stock
2 tbsp Tomato Puree
225g Risotto Rice
125ml Red Wine
1½tbsp Plant-Based Butter
Salt
Black Pepper

Mix It Up:

To be honest, you don't want to change a thing about this dish. It is that good!

RATATOUILLE RISOTTO (VE, GF, DF)

Recipe:

1. Trim the aubergine, courgette, and tomatoes, cut them into 2cm chunks, and place them on a lined baking tray. Drizzle with 2 tbsp of olive oil and season with salt and black pepper. Put in a pre-heated oven (200°C or 180°C fan assisted) for 40 minutes.

2. Peel and finely chop the red onion, garlic, and sundried tomatoes. Place the stock in a saucepan on low heat.

3. Warm the remaining olive oil in a frying pan over medium heat. Add the onion and cook for 10-15 minutes until soft and translucent. Peel and mince the garlic, add to the pan and cook for a further minute. Then add the rosemary, thyme, sun-dried tomatoes, and tomato puree. Give everything a good stir and cook for 4 – 5 minutes.

4. Add the rice and stir for a minute. Turn up the heat slightly, add the red wine and then stir until the rice absorbs it. Add the stock a ladle at a time, waiting until the stock is absorbed before adding the next ladleful.

5. After about 15 minutes, the rice should be about 3 minutes away from being al dente. Take the roasted ratatouille vegetables out of the oven, scrape them into the pan, and fold them into the risotto. Continue to stir until the rice cooks. Remove from the heat and then stir in the butter. Finally, season with salt and black pepper.

CAULIFLOWER STEW (VE, GF, DF)

Estimated Time: 75 minutes

Serves: 4

This Greek-inspired dish proves that you can create a vegan masterpiece for any occasion, even Sunday lunch.

Equipment:	Ingredients:
Speed Peeler	1 Lemon
Tablespoon	2 tbsp Olive Oil
Large Casserole Pan with Lid	1 Garlic Bulb
Chopping Board	2 Red Onions
Large Kitchen Knife	10 Black Olives
Tablespoon	300g New Potatoes
Wooden Spoon	15g Fresh Oregano
Kettle	10 Plum Tomatoes
Measuring Jug	1 Head of Cauliflower
Fork	200g Frozen Peas
	500ml Water

Mix It Up:

Try some frozen broad or runner beans instead of peas, and give leeks a go to provide a different flavour.

CAULIFLOWER STEW (VE, GF, DF)

Recipe:

1. Use a speed peeler to strip the lemon zest into a large casserole pan on medium heat. Add the oil and the whole garlic bulb.

2. Peel and quarter the onions and separate the petals before adding to the pan. Destone the olives and add to the pan. Scrub the potatoes and cut them into 1 cm thick slices. Add them to the pan, along with the oregano leaves. Cook for 5 minutes, and then quarter and add the tomatoes.

3. Pour in the water and bring to a boil. Stir well, scraping the sticky bits from the bottom of the pan. Remove the cauliflower's outer leaves. Then cut a small cross in the stalk before pushing it right down into the pan. Drizzle it with a tablespoon of olive oil, cover the pan, and then put in a preheated oven (220°C or 200°C fan assisted) for an hour. Baste the cauliflower regularly and remove the lid for the final 30 minutes.

4. Once cooked, remove the cauliflower to a plate and pick out the garlic bulb. Add the pan back to heat and add the frozen peas and simmer for 5 minutes. Using a fork, carefully squeeze all the garlic from the roasted cloves and add it to the pan. Slice the cauliflower into four and place on plates. Then add lemon juice to the vegetable mix and serve alongside the cauliflower.

RAINBOW STIR FRY (VE, GF, DF)

Estimated Time: 25 minutes

Serves: 4

Quite possibly the best stir fry ever! With so many varied ingredients, you get a different flavour burst with every mouthful.

Equipment:

Chopping Board
Large Kitchen Knife
Tablespoon
Blender
Wooden Spoon
Large Wok
Fine Grater
Bowl
Kitchen Scales

Ingredients:

3 Garlic Cloves
3 Limes
1-2 Red Chillies
1 tbsp Soy Sauce
1½ tbsp Rice Wine Vinegar
30g Fresh Coriander
1 Red Onion
5cm Piece of Ginger
1 Red Pepper
40g Cavolo Nero
50g Tenderstem Broccoli
50g Baby Sweetcorn
1 Carrot
50g Frozen Broad Beans
150g Rice Noodles
½ tbsp Olive Oil
1 tsp Sesame Oil
60g Mangetout
25g Cashews
Salt
Black Pepper

RAINBOW STIR FRY (VE, GF, DF)

Recipe:

1. First, make the sauce. Peel the garlic and deseed the chillies. Roughly chop both and place in a blender, along with the soy sauce, vinegar, lime juice, and 20g of coriander. Blitz until smooth.

2. Next, prep the veg. Peel and thinly slice the red onion. Peel and grate the ginger. Trim, halve, and core the red pepper, then cut thinly into strips. Remove the centre stalk from the cavolo nero and roughly chop the leaves. Trim and quarter the broccoli, halve the baby sweetcorn lengthways, peel the carrot and cut it into matchsticks. Then cook the broad beans as per instructions.

3. Thinly slice the radishes and spring onion, setting them aside for later. Cook the noodles as per packet instructions. Drain and return to a bowl, add the sauce and then toss to combine.

4. Pour the oil into a wok (or large frying pan) over high heat. Firstly, add the red onion, ginger, pepper, and a pinch of salt. As you continuously stir, add the additional ingredients as follows. After one minute, throw in the broccoli and sweetcorn, and then after a further 60 seconds, the cavolo nero, beans, and sesame oil. Stir in the carrot and mangetout before finally adding the prepared noodles.

5. Place the cooked stir fry in a bowl or on a plate and top with the remaining coriander leaves, some roughly chopped cashews, and serve with a lime wedge.

VEGGIE PAD THAI (V, GF, DF)

Estimated Time: 25 minutes

Serves: 4

This delicious national dish was created in the 1930s by Thai prime minister Plaek Phibunsongkhram.

Equipment:

2 Bowls
Teaspoon
2 Frying Pans
Electric Mini Chopper
Garlic Press
Fork
Chopping Board
Large Kitchen Knife
Tablespoon
Kitchen Scales

Ingredients:

200g Rice Noodles
2 tsp Sesame Oil
20g Unsalted Peanuts
2 Garlic Cloves
80g Silken Tofu
1 tbsp Soy Sauce
2 tsp Tamarind Paste
2 tsp Sweet Chilli Sauce
2 Limes
1 Large Shallot
400g Crunchy Veg (Asparagus, Broccoli, Baby Sweetcorn or Pak Choi)
80g Beansprouts
4 Eggs
Olive Oil
Chilli Flakes
Cos Lettuce
15g of Mixed Fresh Herbs (Mint, Basil and Coriander)

VEGGIE PAD THAI (V, GF, DF)

Recipe:

1. Cook the noodles to packet instructions, drain, and refresh with cold water before tossing in a bowl with the sesame oil. Toast the peanuts, in a small frying pan, over medium heat, and then blitz until fine using the mini chopper. Set aside both for later.

2. Peel and mince the garlic. Add to a bowl, along with the tofu, then add one teaspoon of sesame oil, soy sauce, tamarind paste, and chilli sauce. Mash into a paste using the back of a fork. Muddle in half the juice of the lime and a splash of water to loosen the mixture.

3. Peel and finely slice the shallot and place in a frying pan over high heat. Trim, prep, and cut the crunchy veg as necessary, and then add to the pan and dry fry for 4 minutes. Add the noodles, sauce, beansprouts, and another good splash of water. Toss the ingredients together over the heat for a minute and then divide between the plates, serving the noodle mix on top of a few Cos lettuce leaves.

4. Wipe the pan, add some olive oil and then cook the eggs to your liking. Pop the eggs on top of the noodles and sprinkle with a pinch of chilli flakes. Serve with lime wedges for squeezing over and a little soy sauce if needed.

BUTTER CHICKPEA CURRY (V, GF, DF)

Estimated Time: 30 minutes

Serves: 4

This Indian Butter Curry has a silky-smooth texture and just enough spicy kick to create a warm sensation inside.

Equipment:

Chopping Board
Large Kitchen Knife
Tablespoon
Large Frying Pan
Wooden Spoon
Fine Grater
Measuring Jug
Saucepan

Ingredients:

2 tbsp Butter
400g Chickpeas
1 Onion
2 tsp Garam Masala
2 tsp Ground Coriander
2 tsp Ground Cumin
2 tsp Ground Turmeric
1 Garlic Clove
4cm Fresh Ginger
1 tbsp Tomato Puree
400ml Passata
200ml Coconut Milk
Salt
Black Pepper
Olive Oil
1 Green Chilli
10g Fresh Coriander
Basmati Rice and / or Naans

Mix It Up:

Try tofu or butter beans rather than chickpeas. Crank up the heat with a scotch bonnet chilli.

BUTTER CHICKPEA CURRY (V, GF, DF)

Recipe:

1. Melt one tablespoon of butter in a large frying pan over medium heat. Peel and roughly chop the onion and add to the pan with a pinch of salt, cooking for 3-4 minutes. Add the spices and cook for 1 minute.

2. Peel the garlic and ginger and grate them both directly into the pan. Add the tomato puree and cook for 2 minutes. Pour in the passata, bring to the boil and then reduce the heat to a simmer for 10 minutes.

3. Cook the basmati rice as per packet instructions.

4. Drain the chickpeas, if necessary, and set them aside.

5. Add the coconut milk and the remaining butter to the sauce, season with salt and black pepper, and then stir in the chickpeas. Leave to simmer for 5 minutes, allowing the chickpeas to heat through.

6. Heat through the naans, if using, and then serve alongside the rice and curry. Finely slice the green chilli and coriander, sprinkling on top of the curry.

PAELLA (VE, GF, DF)

Estimated Time: 70 minutes

Serves: 4

This dish is simply brilliant as it comes and is well worth the time and attention to cook it!

Equipment:

Chopping Board
Large Kitchen Knife
Tablespoon
Frying Pan or Paella Pan
Wooden Spoon
Saucepan for the Stock
Measuring Jug
Ladle
Kitchen Foil
2 Tea Towels
Kitchen Scales

Ingredients:

1 Roasted Red Pepper
200g Butter Beans
1 Onion
1 Garlic Clove
1 Tomato
150g Green Beans
200g Tenderstem Broccoli
200g Artichoke Hearts
Pinch of Saffron
1 tbsp Olive Oil
1 tbsp Paprika
½ tsp Ground Turmeric
1l Veg Stock
280g Paella Rice
1-2 Lemons
Salt
Black Pepper

PAELLA (VE, GF, DF)

Recipe:

1. Cut the roasted pepper in half, and cut the flesh into 1½ cm strips. Reserve 5 strips, and chop the rest into smaller pieces. Drain the butter beans, peel and finely chop the onion, garlic, and tomato. Trim the green beans and cut the heads off the broccoli. Cut the beans and broccoli stems into 1-2 cm pieces. Quarter the artichoke hearts. Set aside all the chopped veg.

2. Heat the olive oil in a frying pan over medium heat. Add the onions and cook for 10 minutes, and then add the garlic, stirring for a couple of minutes. Add the tomato and cook for a further 10 minutes, then stir in the saffron, paprika, turmeric, and a generous pinch of salt and black pepper. Add the stock to the pan and bring to the boil, then reduce to medium heat.

3. Stir in the green beans, tenderstem stalks, butter beans, artichokes, and red pepper pieces (reserving the strips). Increase to boil, then turn down to medium and simmer. Sprinkle the rice evenly over the pan, bring to the boil again, reduce to medium, and simmer without stirring for 5 mins. Add the pepper strips and tenderstem heads to the surface, and cook without stirring for 10 minutes.

4. After 10 minutes, the rice should be translucent but al dente. If the pan starts to dry out during the 10 minutes, simply add 100ml boiling water, slowly using a ladle. Once the time has expired, turn up the heat to give it a blast to remove any liquid. Remove from the heat and

cover the pan with foil and two tea towels. Leave it for 10-15 mins, as this improves the taste and texture. Then cut the lemon into wedges and serve alongside the paella.

Thank you for the inspiration.

Veggie Lean in 15 by Joe Wicks
California Scramble
Spring Onion, Spinach and Cheese Frittata
Spicy Halloumi Burger and Sweet Potato Fries
BBQ Sweet Potato Quesadillas
Huevos Rancheros
Paella

BOSH! by Henry Firth & Ian Theasby
Portobello Mushroom Burger and Rosemary Fries
Ratatouille Risotto

BOSH! Healthy Vegan by Henry Firth & Ian Theasby
Mushroom Caesar Salad
Rainbow Stir Fry

Speedy BOSH! by Henry Firth & Ian Theasby
Breakfast Hash Tacos
Butter Chickpea Curry

VEG by Jamie Oliver
Asparagus, Potato and Leek Soup
Cauliflower Stew
Veggie Pad Thai

The Hairy Dieters Go Veggie by Si King and Dave Myers
Creamed Spinach with Eggs

The Greek Vegetarian Cookbook by Heather Thomas
One Pan Brunch

APPENDIX II: THE EXERCISES

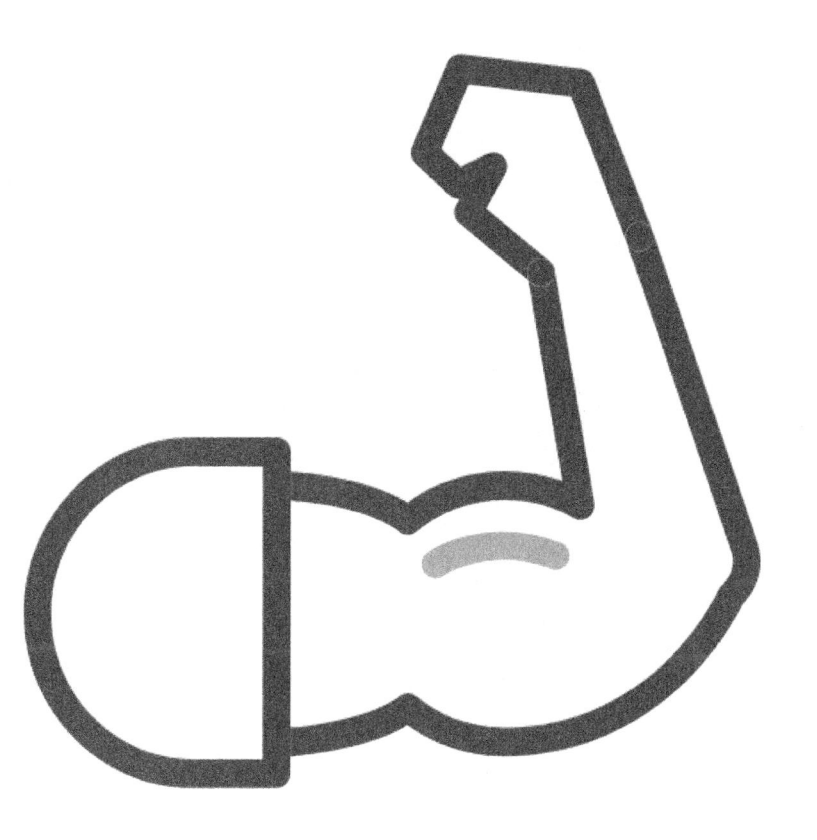

STRETCHING EXERCISES

Hip Flexor

Starting on your hands and knees, place your hands directly under your shoulders and step your feet out behind you, with your feet hip-width apart. Your arms should be at 90º to the floor and keep your head, neck, upper body, and legs in a straight line. Bring your left foot up, placing it outside your left hand. Hold the position for a few seconds before returning to the starting position. Repeat with your right foot.

Hamstring

Sit on the floor with your legs extended in front. Raise both arms above your head, breathe in, and then lower your hands towards your feet. Hinge at the waist and keep your back as straight as possible. Hold for ten seconds, then return to the starting position before repeating. As a beginner, you may only reach your knees or shins.

Downward Dog

Start on all fours, with your hands shoulder-width apart and fingers spread wide. Press your hands into the mat, and take a deep breath. Continue to press your hands into the mat, exhale, and lift your knees away from the ground. Straighten your legs as much as possible, pushing your heels into, or as close to, the ground as possible. Keep your tailbone up. Keep your back long from the tailbone to the back of the head.

Cobra (Upward Dog)

Lie face down on the floor, with your hands next to your shoulders, and your legs stretched out. Lift your upper body away from the floor, keeping a slight bend at the elbow. If you wish to advance the move, then twist your head to the left, looking over your shoulder, and then repeat to the right.

Chest Extension

Stand upright with your feet shoulder-width apart. Lift your arms out in front, perpendicular to the shoulders. Open your arms as if you are stretching an elastic band. Extend as far as is comfortable before returning your arms to the starting position. You can change the angles slightly by opening your arms at 45°, either above or below shoulder height.

Quad

Lie on your left side with your legs straight and knees together. Pull your right foot to your glute (bum) with your right hand. Hold for ten seconds and then repeat with your left foot while lying on your right side.

Glute

Sit on the floor with your legs extended in front. Bend your right knee, and plant your right foot to the outside of your left knee. Using both forearms, pull your right knee towards your chest until you feel a pull in your glute. Do not overextend the knee as this can cause discomfort. Hold for ten seconds before swapping to the other side.

Lateral

Stand upright with your arms above your head and your palms together. Stretch upwards and then lean to the left, holding for five seconds, feeling the stretch in your side, before returning to the starting position. Repeat the stretch, this time leaning to the right.

Triceps

Raise your left arm over your head. Bend at the elbow, so your left hand is behind your neck. Stretch the back of your left upper arm by pulling your left elbow towards your head with your right hand. Hold for ten seconds and then repeat with the right arm.

Walkout

Stand with your legs in a wide stance. Bending at the waist, place your hand on the floor and walk them out into the press-up position. Walk your hands back and then stand up straight. To increase the intensity, you can complete a press-up before walking the hands back.

CARDIO EXERCISES

Press Up

Starting on your hands and knees, place your hands directly under your shoulders and step your feet out, with your feet hip-width apart. Ensure your arms are at 90° to the floor and your head, neck, upper body, and legs are in a straight line. Lower your body towards the ground, and as your chest reaches the ground, press your body up, extending your arms fully. You can add variation by placing your hands narrower and pushing from the knees rather than the feet.

Running On The Spot

Stand with feet hip-width apart. As you run on the spot, lift your opposite knee and arm. Lift the knees as high as possible and your hands to at least shoulder height. You can add variation by punching out or lifting your arms above your head (as if pulling down on a rope).

Squats

Stand with your feet shoulder-width apart. Hold your arms out in front and slowly lower into the squat. You should keep your head up, back straight as you lower, and knees directly over your feet. Once your thighs are parallel to the ground, pause, then raise yourself back into the starting position. You can add variation by taking your feet wider into a sumo-style squat.

Burpees

Stand with your feet hip-width apart. Drop into a squat and place your hands on the floor. Kick your legs out so that you are in the press-up position. Bring your legs back in, and then jump up with your hands above your head. Land softly and repeat.

Mountain Climbers

Set yourself in the press-up position. Alternate bringing each knee towards your chest. Increase your speed for higher intensity, or walk your feet in and out if you are a beginner.

Star Jumps

Stand upright with your feet together and arms at your side. Jump your feet out laterally, simultaneously raising your arms above the head. Your arms and legs should form a star shape. Jump back to the starting position and repeat.

Squat Thrust

Starting in the press-up position, jump both feet in, bringing your knees towards your chest. Then kick out both legs back into the press-up position and repeat.

Press Up Jack
Starting in the press-up position, jump both feet out laterally, as far as you feel comfortable. Jump back into the starting position. For added intensity, you can alternate between press-up jacks and squat thrusts.

Lateral Jumps
Stand with your feet hip-width apart and lower into a shallow squat. Explosively hop off both feet and move to your right. Land softly into a squat and immediately hop back to the left.

Squat Jumps With Shuffle Back
Stand with your feet hip-width apart and lower into a shallow squat. Dip your knees, then explosively hop off both feet and move forward. Land softly into a squat and immediately hop forward again. Land softly, stand, and shuffle back to the start point.

ABS EXERCISES

Plank
Starting on your hands and knees, place your hands directly under your shoulders and step your feet out. Ensure you keep your back in a straight line and not dipped or raised. You can add variation by placing your forearms on the floor with your elbows directly below your shoulders. Breathe steadily throughout.

Side Plank
Lie on your side with your legs straight. Lift onto your forearm, which should be perpendicular to your body.

Ensure your shoulder is directly above your elbow. Raise your other arm in the air. Breathe steadily throughout.

Crunches

Lie on your back with your knees bent and your feet flat on the floor. Place your hands on your thighs, and then curl forward, keeping your eyes skyward, so your head, neck, and shoulder blades lift off the floor while sliding your hands to your knees. Hold for a moment and then slowly lower back down, keeping your eyes skyward at all times. Exhale as you crunch up and inhale as you lower.

Leg Raises

Lie on your back with your legs straight and your arms at your side. Raise both legs so they are perpendicular to the floor. Lift your shoulder blades off the floor, and slowly lower both legs. Just before your feet touch the floor, raise both legs back to the starting point. Inhale as you lower and exhale as you lift your legs.

Reverse Crunches

Lie on your back with your knees bent and your feet flat on the floor. Place your hands at your side. Raise both legs, curling your knees to your chest, lifting your hips off the floor. Slowly lower your legs to the starting position. Exhale as you curl your knees to your chest and inhale as you lower.

Toe Touches

Lie on your back with your legs straight. Raise both your arms and legs so that they are perpendicular to the floor. Curl upward, raising your shoulder blades off the floor and moving your fingers towards your toes. Exhale as you curl upwards and inhale as you lower.

Knee To Elbow

Starting on your hands and knees, place your hands directly under your shoulders and step your feet out. Slowly bring your left knee toward your left elbow. Return to the starting position before repeating with your right knee moving towards your right elbow. You can add variation by placing your forearms on the floor, with your elbows directly below your shoulders. Breathe steadily throughout.

Bicycle Crunches

Lie on your back with your legs straight. Place your hands on the side of your head and lift your shoulder blades off the floor. Raise both legs slightly, and then bring the left knee in towards your chest. As you complete this move, twist at the waist to bring the right elbow towards the knee. Lower both the leg and arm while simultaneously bring the opposite limbs together. Breathe steadily throughout.

Flutter Kicks

Lie on your back with your legs straight and your arms at your side. Raise both legs so they are 6 to 12 inches off the ground. Lift your shoulder blades off the floor, and flick your feet up and down, moving them no more than 1 to 2 inches. Breathe steadily throughout.

V Twist

Lie on your back with your knees bent and your feet flat on the floor. Lift your upper body so that it is as close to 45° to the floor as possible. From this position, twist your upper body, alternately from left to right. Allow your arms to follow the motion as if moving a box from side to side.

DUMBBELL EXERCISES

Bicep Curls
Stand upright, with your feet shoulder-width apart. Hold one dumbbell in each hand, relax your arms down to the side, with your palms facing inwards. Keep your upper arms stable and relax your shoulders. Lift the dumbbells, bending and twisting at the elbows, until the weights are at shoulder height. Ensure you move at a steady pace, keeping your elbows tucked into your upper body. Inhale as you lower and exhale as you raise.

Triceps Extensions
Stand with your feet shoulder-width apart. Hold a dumbbell in each hand, bend forward at the waist so your upper body is almost parallel to the floor. Your arm should be at 90º to your upper body. Engage your core and keep your head, neck, and spine in a straight line. Slowly extend your lower arms back as far as you can, keeping your upper arms tucked into your upper body. Exhale as you extend and inhale as you contract your arms.

Shoulder Press
Stand with your feet slightly wider than shoulder-width apart. Holding a dumbbell in each hand, lift them to shoulder height, with your palms facing forward. Slowly raise both arms above your head and slowly return to shoulder height. Exhale as you press and then inhale as you lower.

Bent-Over Row
Stand with your feet shoulder-width apart. Hold a dumbbell in each hand with your palms facing the body. Bend over from the waist at no more than 45º, with a slight bend in the knees, and keeping your back straight. Lift the

dumbbells straight up, ensuring the arms do not go above shoulder height and then lower in a controlled manner. Exhale as you raise the dumbbells and inhale as you lower.

Floor To Ceiling

Stand upright with your feet slightly narrower than hip-width apart. Hold a dumbbell in each hand, at the side of the body, and with your palms facing inwards. Slowly squat, taking the dumbbells toward the ground, allowing them to kiss the floor at your side. Then as you raise out of the squat, curl the dumbbells up to the shoulders. Press the dumbbells overhead, palms facing inwards. Exhale on the upward movement and inhale as you drop back into the squat.

KETTLEBELL EXERCISES

Swing

Stand with your feet wider than shoulder-width apart and your knees slightly bent. Holding the kettlebell with both hands, and keeping your arms straight, swing it in a pendulum motion, from just below the groin up to eye level. Exhale as you swing up and inhale as the kettlebell returns to the start point.

Reverse Lunge

Stand upright with your feet together, your back straight, and holding the kettlebell close to your chest. Step backward, bending the back leg at the knee. The knee should nearly touch the ground. Your front knee should bend so your thigh is parallel to the floor. Step back into the starting position and alternate. Inhale as you enter the lunge, and exhale as you return to the standing position.

Squat With Shoulder Press
Stand with your feet slightly wider than shoulder-width apart. Hold the kettlebell in one hand, level with the shoulder, and slowly lower into a squat position. Power up out of the squat and press the kettlebell overhead, straightening your arm completely. Return the kettlebell to shoulder level and repeat. Once your repetitions are complete, repeat with the other arm. Inhale as you lower into the squat and exhale as you power out.

Romanian Dead Lift
Stand with your feet shoulder-width apart, holding a kettlebell with both hands in front of your legs. Plant both feet on the floor and bend your knees slightly. Bending from the hips, lower the kettlebell towards to ground until you feel the tension in your hamstring. Use your glutes and hamstrings to return to the starting position. Inhale as you lower and exhale as you raise.

Goblet Squat
Place your feet in a wide stance holding the kettlebell close to your chest. Keep your back straight, and lower slowly into the squat. Hold the squat and then slowly rise back to the starting position. Inhale as you lower, then exhale as you raise.

WORKOUTS

These workouts follow the principles of high-intensity interval training. If you are new to this type of training, start with the shortest duration before building toward more intense workouts.

You can choose a combination of exercises from each of the four categories; cardio, abs, dumbbell, or kettlebell, or stick with one type only. Here are a couple of examples using the workouts for beginners, where you have to complete 15 exercises in total.

Workout One

You choose five exercises from one category and then repeat each one three times, for example.

Dumbbell: Bicep Curls, Tricep Extensions, Shoulder Press, Bent-Over Row, Floor to Ceiling

Workout Two

You choose five exercises from three different categories, for example.

Cardio: Press Up, Running on the Spot, Squats, Burpees, Mountain Climbers
Abs: Plank, Crunches, Toe Touches, Flutter Kicks, Bicycle Crunches
Kettlebell: Swing, Reverse Lunge, Squat with Shoulder Press, Romanian Deadlift, Goblet Squat

Beginners

Duration: 15 minutes
Work and Rest: 30 seconds work, 30 seconds rest
Workout One: Five different exercises for three rounds
Workout Two: 15 different exercises for one round

Intermediate

Duration: 20 minutes
Work and Rest: 35 seconds work, 25 seconds rest
Workout One: Five different exercises for four rounds
Workout Two: 10 different exercises for two rounds
Workout Three: 20 different exercises for one round

Advanced

Duration: 25 minutes
Work and Rest: 40 seconds work, 20 seconds rest
Workout One: Five different exercises for five rounds
Workout Two: Six different exercises for four rounds + a 40 seconds plank
Workout Three: Four different exercises for six rounds + a 40 seconds plank
Workout Four: 25 different exercises for one round

Tabata

Duration: 20 minutes

Work and Rest: 20 seconds work, 10 seconds rest

Workout One: 40 different exercises for one round

Workout Two: 20 different exercises for two rounds

Workout Three: 10 different exercises for four rounds

Super Sets (Back to Back Exercises from different categories, e.g., Cardio and Abs)

Duration: 30 minutes

Work and Rest: 90 seconds work (2 x 45 seconds), 15 seconds rest

Workout: 10 exercises (Five Super Sets) for three rounds

ACKNOWLEDGMENTS

In October 2020, I could only have dreamt of writing and publishing a book. Over the following nine months, so many people were directly or indirectly involved in getting Fuelled, Fit and Fired Up into publication.

Firstly, I want to give a massive shout-out to the brilliant Michael Heppell, who not only wrote the book's foreword but provided inspiration, challenge, and support during this project. His Write That Book Masterclass shared knowledge, experience, and insight from leading authors, publishers, and marketing experts, all of which influenced the writing of Fuelled, Fit and Fired Up.

A huge thank you to the members of Team 17, How To Be Brilliant and Write That Book Masterclass, particularly my accountability groups; *The Genuine Article, Step Up Step Out, and The Scribblers*. Their unconditional support, encouragement, and feedback played a significant part in the book you see before you today.

Thank you to my friends who invested their time reading and critiquing my initial drafts, providing invaluable and insightful thoughts on the content.

And finally, a huge thank you to the most important person. YOU, the reader. You have brought my dream of being a published author to life, and for that, I will be eternally grateful.

ABOUT THE AUTHOR

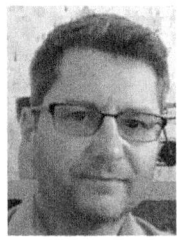

DAVID ROGERS is a strategic business leader who has worked for over 25 years in the private sector. Having spent the last 15 years in the Hospitality sector, he has developed a people-focused passion for wellbeing and personal development. By coupling this enthusiasm with a natural curiosity, his goal is to deliver positive experiences to everyone he meets.

Outside of work, he coaches, mentors, and advises schools and students on their career development strategies. He is an advocate for community projects and is currently a Board Trustee for a charity providing outreach services to vulnerable residents.

Originally from Dudley, in the West Midlands, he now resides in Wombourne, a large village in South Staffordshire, with his wife Amanda and three dogs. He enjoys reading, cooking healthy food, and keeping fit.

Born from his desire to change, Fuelled, Fit and Fired Up is a vehicle to share his learning through simple ideas and practical techniques. He aims to help others improve their personal and professional lives through health, fitness, and wellbeing.

SOCIAL MEDIA

If you want to follow Fuelled, Fit and Fired Up on social media, then you can find me here:

Facebook: @fuelledfitandfiredup
https://www.facebook.com/fuelledfitandfiredup

Instagram: @fuelledfitandfiredup
https://www.instagram.com/fuelledfitandfiredup/

Twitter: @FuelledFitFired
https://twitter.com/FuelledFitFired

If you would like to connect with the author on LinkedIn
https://www.linkedin.com/in/davidneilrogers/